DREAMS

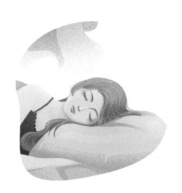

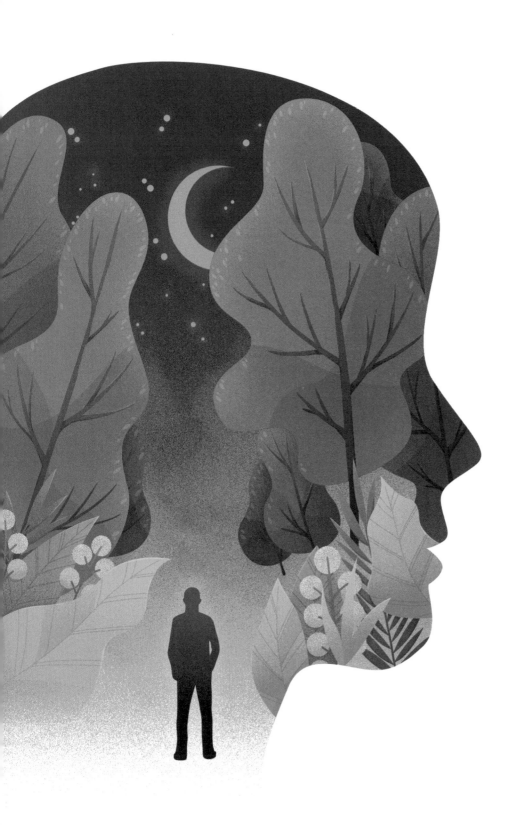

DREAMS

Unlock inner wisdom, discover meaning, and refocus your life

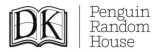

Senior Editor Emma Hill
Senior Art Editor Karen Constanti
US Editor Kayla Dugger
Designer Amy Child
Editorial Assistant Kiron Gill
Senior Jacket Creative Nicola Powling
Jackets Coordinator Lucy Philpott
Senior Producer (Pre-production)
Tony Phipps
Senior Producer Luca Bazzoli
Creative Technical Support
Sonia Charbonnier
Managing Editor Dawn Henderson
Managing Art Editor Marianne Markham
Art Director Maxine Pedliham
Publishing Director Mary-Clare Jerram

Illustrated by Weitong Mai

First American Edition, 2019
Published in the United States by DK Publishing
1450 Broadway, Suite 801, New York, NY 10018

Copyright © 2019 Dorling Kindersley Limited
DK, a Division of Penguin Random House LLC
19 20 21 22 23 10 9 8 7 6 5 4 3 2 1
001–312772–Oct/2019

A catalog record for this book
is available from the Library of Congress.
ISBN 978-1-4654-8241-9

Printed and bound in China

A WORLD OF IDEAS:
SEE ALL THERE IS TO KNOW

www.dk.com

CONTENTS

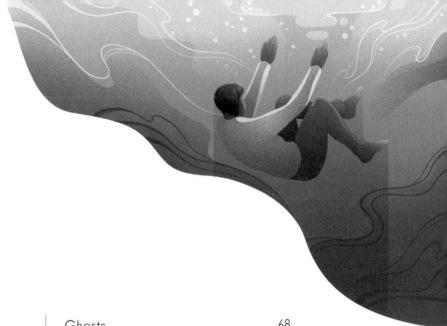

Continued »

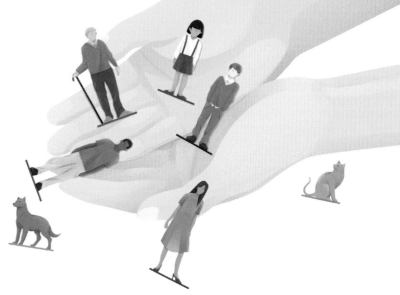

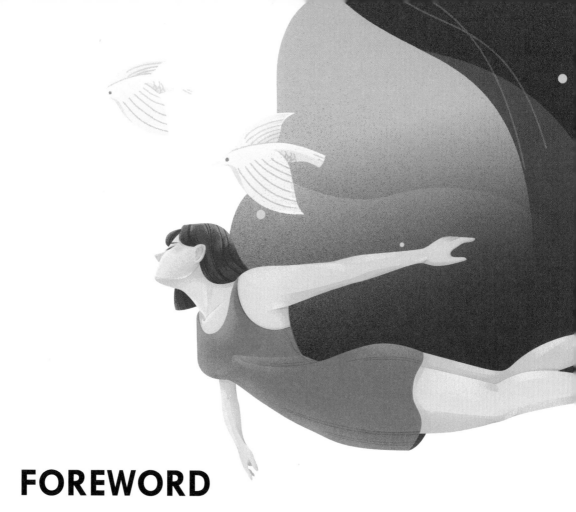

FOREWORD

Dreams are our allies. They are magical friends that teach us about who we are and why we are here, even if they sometimes appear as nightmares. They have been known to trace long-lost friends from thousands of miles away, to predict where people are going to live, and to give advice with a wisdom beyond the dreamer's conscious mind. And yet most people claim they seldom dream—besides, aren't they all just garbage?

Making sense of dreams is undeniably for most people a difficult, if not impossible, task. This book is designed to help decode the more common ones and to point readers toward a clearer understanding of how the psyche works. But dream interpretation is essentially nonscientific: one size does not fit all. Many factors must be considered, and these pages are here to introduce and hopefully encourage you to pursue your interest.

Dreams seem to cooperate only when they deem it's the right time. This does not come from some haughty hierarchy of power, with psyche in control over conscious mind, yet we must respect their dominion—the dream world is not to be commanded or taken lightly.

As you will discover, the messages—often delivered through the medium of metaphor or

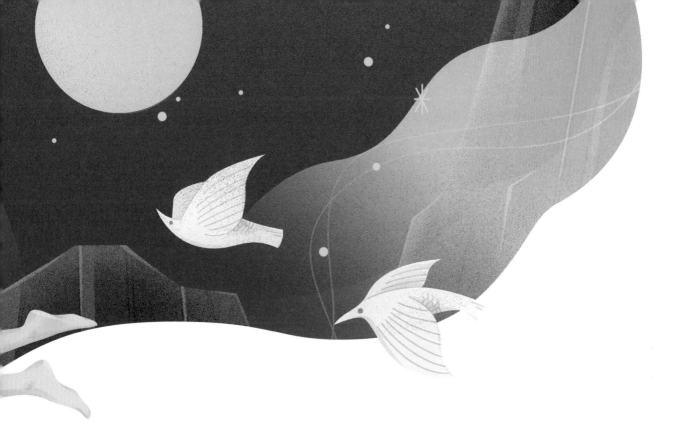

symbols—are the most intriguing aspect of dreams. Why do they arrive, astute and to the point? Why in metaphors? Consider the practice of ancient teachers: they told stories almost exclusively in this way, helping followers understand important concepts by offering verbal pictures to explain their meaning. Dreams seem to follow the same format: always our wise teacher, however confusing they can sometimes seem at first. Reflection later is invaluable, and this is where The Dream Directory should help steer your thinking.

Life today is hard—if not alarming—as we contemplate global warming, political chaos, and an upsurge in mental and physical distress worldwide. People are increasingly turning inward to try to get in touch with guidance so sadly lacking out there. Through studying your dreams, interpreting wherever possible the extraordinary overview our psyches clearly possess, you might learn and discover what else lies waiting for exploration in those hidden realms.

Rosie March Smith

THE THEORY
OF DREAMS

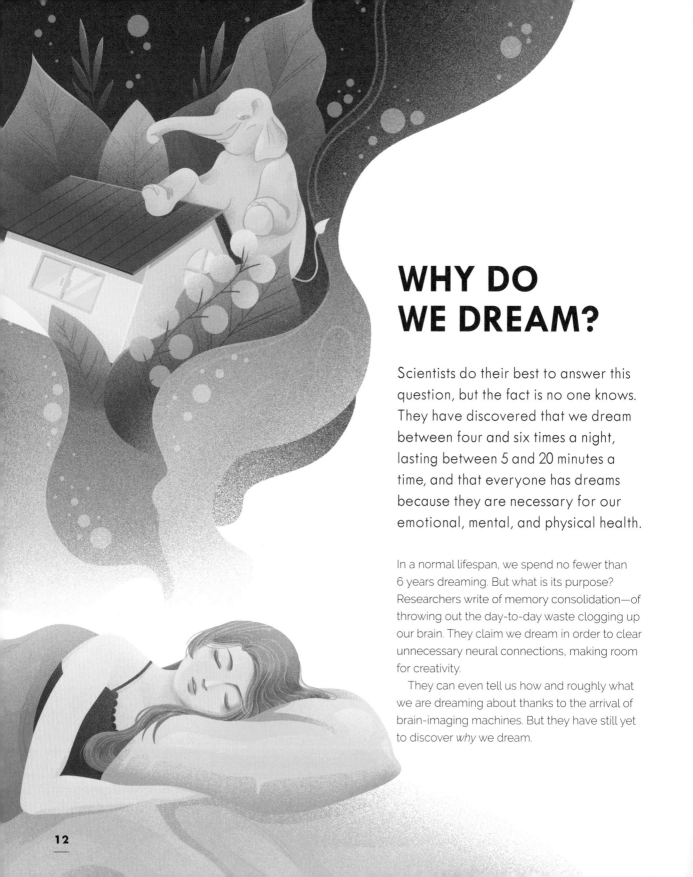

WHY DO WE DREAM?

Scientists do their best to answer this question, but the fact is no one knows. They have discovered that we dream between four and six times a night, lasting between 5 and 20 minutes a time, and that everyone has dreams because they are necessary for our emotional, mental, and physical health.

In a normal lifespan, we spend no fewer than 6 years dreaming. But what is its purpose? Researchers write of memory consolidation—of throwing out the day-to-day waste clogging up our brain. They claim we dream in order to clear unnecessary neural connections, making room for creativity.

They can even tell us how and roughly what we are dreaming about thanks to the arrival of brain-imaging machines. But they have still yet to discover *why* we dream.

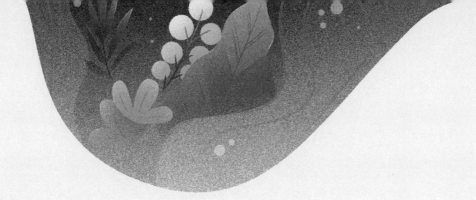

A link to the collective unconscious

Dreams are a conduit to the higher and deeper realms of the mind. If you imagine an island with only its hills and peaks showing above the ocean, it represents symbolically the depth and width of our unconscious world. Next, imagine that ocean bed going, as it does, right around the globe and appreciate how it must connect with everything. This is the basis for Carl Jung's theory of the collective unconscious, where we are all somehow connected. Psychics say this linking mind energy lies behind their clairvoyant ability, privy to the wholeness of our world.

Undoubtedly, quantum physicists are now coming up with fascinating research into "outside time," which could perhaps definitively lead to an answer to the great mysteries.

Dreams as messages

Most traditional rationalists are at a loss to explain how it is that people can dream accurately about their own personal future. They go weeks without remembering any nighttime scenario, then suddenly a vivid, prescient message from the unknown surprises them.

Dream messages and precognition have been recorded for thousands of years. Could we, at some level, be tapping into information from the collective unconscious, which also existed for our ancient ancestors, seers, and prophets?

If the sacred task of dreams is to help us—without technology's limitations—to make more spiritual sense of those hidden realms of the unconscious, perhaps it is timely to believe they are nudging us forward in this turbulent world to a more holistic way of life.

REM AND NREM SLEEP

Using brainwave technology, researchers discovered that dreaming occurs mainly during rapid eye movement (REM) behind closed eyelids. We dream in sleep cycles—sometimes REM, but also nonrapid eye movement (NREM), alternating several times a night. The same may be true of your pets: Have you noticed they twitch in their sleep, as if excited or chasing their prey? Laboratory researchers note a comparable dreaming state in human volunteers, whose heads are wired up to measure brainwave activity, as they move in and out of the respective cycles. Any emotional responses to the dream narrative are clearly traced to synchronize with the electrooculography (EOG) measure, but technology is unable to decipher the dream content.

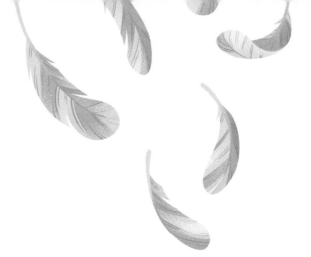

WHAT IS HEALTHY SLEEP?

Most adults sleep between 7 and 9 hours a night. It may seem like a long time out of your day not to be working, running errands, or having fun, but these hours are essential to your health and well-being.

Sleeping well means you safeguard your entire system—body, mind, and spirit. It increases your levels of energy and helps you to think efficiently. It also improves your immune function for fighting, for example, the common cold. More importantly, a regular good night's sleep protects your cardiovascular system, blood sugar levels, and propensity to stress, decreasing your chances of seriously disabling conditions such as heart attacks and strokes. So a good night's rest is crucial for a whole range of health reasons. Unfortunately, there are certain sleep disorders that can negatively impact our ability to form or maintain healthy sleep patterns.

Nightmares

When we think of nightmares, they are usually of the fear-based kind young children confront in their sleep—open as they are to new impressions and bewildering input throughout each day. Monsters and frightening ghosts in the closet are paradoxically helpful: children learn in time that monsters don't exist and that they've conquered their fears—another step toward self-confidence.

But adults experience nightmares as well. Usually appearing in the first hour or so in the NREM phase of sleep, these are of a different nature, caused by serious reality. Posttraumatic stress disorder (PTSD) often lies behind persistent nightmares. Mental illness of all kinds and substance abuse can cause a variety of sleep disorders, from disturbing nightmares to insomnia. For example, schizophrenia involves distortion of perception, delusions, and hallucinations as part of the pattern, which can lead to dreams with similar distortions. And too much alcohol—however initially relaxing—affects the quality of sleep, even to the point of insomnia. Prescribed sleeping tablets can also affect the real advantages of sleep. Some of those drugs interfere with the circadian rhythm and prevent the sleeper from reaching REM (rapid eye movement) and benefiting from the healing quality of deep sleep.

Recurring dreams

Recurring dreams are another aspect of the disorder spectrum, as they are distressing when predictably unpleasant. If the conscious mind has not fully processed past emotional trauma, anger, grief, or fearful episodes, then the unconscious mind will keep replaying it.
It is as if that hidden world of the psyche is trying unsuccessfully to get the message through to consciousness.

It will keep repeating unless those powerful emotions are released from their trapped state, usually by therapy.

CIRCADIAN RHYTHM

Your circadian rhythm is a 24-hour body clock that functions on a regular cycle of alertness and drowsiness. This means during the day—think postlunch snooze—as well as when you sleep. Vivid or bewildering dreams that occur, for example, at times you've flown halfway around the world or worked night shifts are associated not only with poor-quality sleep, but with unhelpful dreams. Trying to decode them is a thankless task. Why? The blame lies with upset hormones resulting from the interruption of your circadian rhythm. The psyche cannot deliver its subtle messages from the unconscious under these conditions, so it is better to wait for your circadian rhythm to settle back to normal.

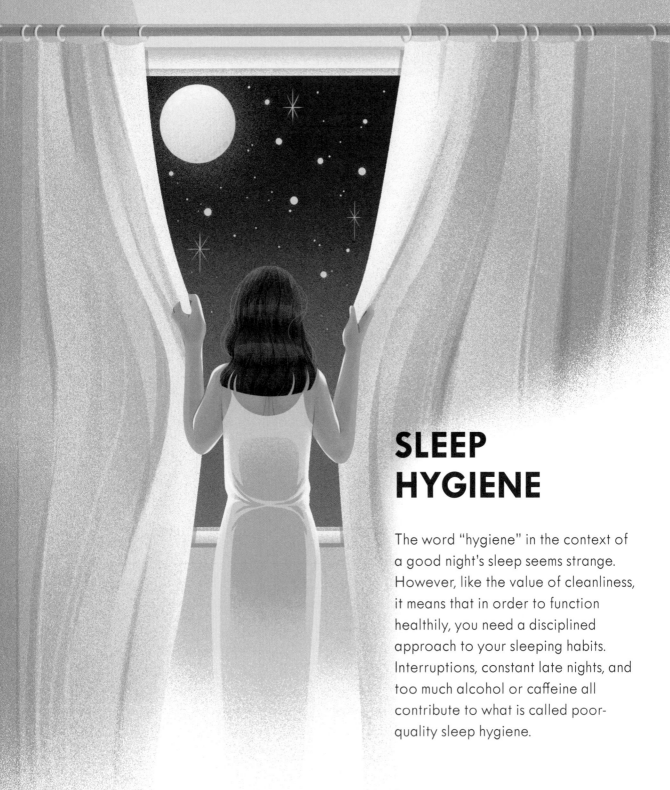

SLEEP HYGIENE

The word "hygiene" in the context of a good night's sleep seems strange. However, like the value of cleanliness, it means that in order to function healthily, you need a disciplined approach to your sleeping habits. Interruptions, constant late nights, and too much alcohol or caffeine all contribute to what is called poor-quality sleep hygiene.

Developing a bedtime routine

Just as babies need to settle into a familiar pattern for bedtime, it's important for you to stick to a regular routine. A growing body of research suggests that the blue light emitted from digital screens prevents your brain from releasing melatonin, which lets your body know when it's time to sleep; therefore, resist scrolling through messages right before bed. Also, avoid having a lively discussion with anyone. You will finish the conversation (or fight) "wired" and have much more difficulty falling asleep.

A book at bedtime can be soothing. A warm bath, yoga, or evening meditation all provide a healthy, relaxing mental space to prepare you for sleep. Worries tend to be more intense when your body and mind are tired from the day's activities, and you are less likely to see them in perspective. Meditation can help push those increasing anxieties away, or at least release tense shoulders and calm a whirring brain.

Creating an optimum setting

Is the room where you sleep comfortable and pleasantly warm without being too warm? A cool 60–65°F (16–18°C) is thought to be the ideal temperature in a bedroom.

If there are bright lights outside your bedroom window at home, put up some blackout material or, better still, use interlined, heavy curtains. If noise is a problem (a snoring partner, perhaps, or traffic hum), a white-noise machine is ideal. You can choose from various models, but ones that offer a choice of background ambient and natural sounds—such as a waterfall or birdsong—can be extraordinarily effective due to their predictable cadences.

THE POWER OF CHEESE

Cheese—usually associated with bad dreams—can be a beneficial aid to a good night's sleep. Cheese contains naturally high levels of tryptophan; from this amino acid, the brain produces serotonin, which is vital for a sense of well-being and happiness. Tryptophan is used to help premenstrual syndrome in women, as well as those suffering from SAD (seasonal affective disorder) or other depressive symptoms, and it is also effective in encouraging restfulness and a good night's sleep. Beyond the fact that really strong, powerfully smelly cheese contains other compounds related to tryptophan that can induce some lively dreams, the old wives' tale about avoiding cheese at bedtime doesn't stand up.

"
WHO LOOKS OUTSIDE, DREAMS; WHO LOOKS INSIDE, AWAKES.

CARL JUNG
MEMORIES, DREAMS, REFLECTIONS

THE DREAM PIONEERS

The ancients knew about dreams—though we glean most through biblical accounts—but it was not until the early 20th century that modern dream interpretation gained a wider understanding. Instead of burning bushes and fiery chariots (which now sound more like UFO sightings than a prophet's warning), dream content held fascinating, intimate details to professional observers. Their significance was seen as profoundly meaningful, revealing at last the inner workings of the dreamer's mind.

Sigmund Freud

Austrian psychiatrist Sigmund Freud, the acknowledged founder of psychoanalysis, ranks as the foremost leader of talk therapy. Freud was the first to recognize the significance of dreams in mental health. He published his book, *The Interpretation of Dreams*, in 1900, setting the stage for psychoanalytic theory and electrifying his colleagues with its daring content: Freud believed his patients' sleep narratives largely held covert sexual conflict.

However, several researchers have wondered since if his own personal struggle with his sexual leanings was not sometimes coloring his interpretations. He insisted that to be accepted by his skeptical peers, it was essential to keep to a strict, rational position. He failed to accept any mystical, otherworldly interpretations suggested by one or two of his students.

Significantly, Freud saw the connection between the tragic Greek character Oedipus—accidentally killing his father and marrying his widowed mother, believing he had been adopted at birth—and the hidden, repressed sexual longings in his patients.

Though he is known mostly today for his theory of repression, Freud developed other important ideas still widely respected over a century later by mental health practitioners.

> "FREUD BELIEVED HIS PATIENTS' SLEEP NARRATIVES LARGELY HELD COVERT SEXUAL CONFLICT."

Continued »

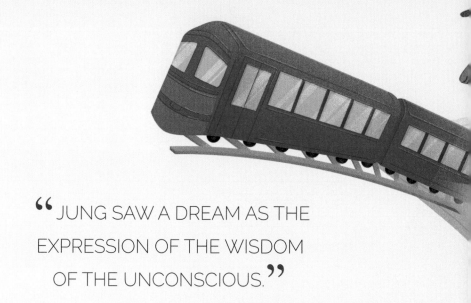

> **"JUNG SAW A DREAM AS THE EXPRESSION OF THE WISDOM OF THE UNCONSCIOUS."**

Carl Jung

An analytical psychologist and Freud's student for some years, Swiss-born Carl Jung's name is synonymous with dream interpretation. Jung has influenced modern dream studies more than anyone. Opposed to his mentor's professed one-track view of dream analysis, Jung broke away, insisting that dreams come from a transcendental source—the world of the spirit. He declared they reflect our waking selves and help solve problems, a far more positive take that contributed to his philosophy that the human psyche has greater influence than personal experience alone.

This led Jung to develop his own ideas about the value of dreams, far removed from hints at the forbidden in disguised form. He saw a dream as the expression of the wisdom of the unconscious. He believed it was often cloaked in symbolism or metaphor, powerfully integrating the conscious with the unconscious—and he valued that concept highly.

Jung saw dreams as useful indicators to determine the dreamer's journey toward individuation: transforming an unformed person into a unique individual. He maintained that women have a masculine (*animus*) side to their psyche while men have a feminine (*anima*) side, both of which are essential for that journey.

Unlike Freud, he embraced the holistic way of life. Jung believed in alchemy, astrology, and mythology. He had the courage to embark on self-analysis to the point of confronting his own unconscious world, considered a dangerous exercise. But as a result of enduring a mental breakdown, he emerged with clear ideas about archetypes, complexes, the collective unconscious, and individuation, all of which still influence psychiatric and psychological teaching today.

Calvin S. Hall

A younger contemporary of Jung, American-born Calvin Springer Hall approached the world of dreams from a different perspective. A behavioral psychologist, he developed a cognitive theory of dreams in the middle of the last century, rejecting Jung's belief that dream content sometimes comes from higher levels

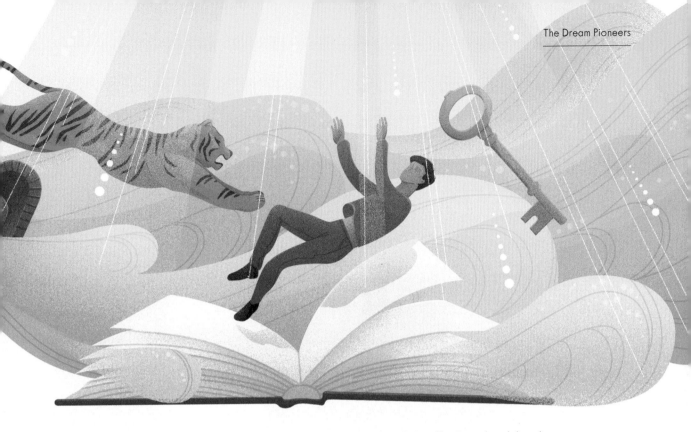

outside the self. He contended they were only the result of the dreamer's personal thoughts, hopes, fears, and experiences.

Hall declared that dreams convey the dreamer's conceptions of self, family, friends, and so on—and that they revealed qualities (for example, "weak," "domineering," or "loving") that essentially mirror the dreamer's own views.

Edgar Cayce

American-born Edgar Cayce, the son of a poor Kentucky farmer, became famous in the early part of the 20th century because of his ability to dream clairvoyantly, diagnosing thousands of grateful patients and—from the sleep state— recommending healing remedies.

The dream world was central to his being. Cayce unwittingly illustrated Jung's idea of group consciousness, demonstrating how he was able to "see" from afar and diagnose unfamiliar people without any prior knowledge

of their condition. But unlike Jung, he claimed to be able to examine trauma in previous lifetimes—as in reincarnation—which frequently explained their present troubles.

Cayce's story began as a boy. He was upset by his father's anger at his difficulty with learning spelling. Once, he laid down with his head on a spelling book and fell fast asleep. Strangely, when he woke up, he knew all the correct answers. Later, he learned in the sleep state how to cure his chronic loss of voice and to heal a long-term boyhood ailment.

Cayce was affectionately known as "The Sleeping Prophet." Thousands of patients over the years asked for his help and valued his "prescriptions"—holistic treatments such as homeopathy, essential oils, mud baths, special diets, and meditation. He used to say "Dreams are tonight's answers to tomorrow's questions," and, like Jung, used symbols to convey meaning to dreams.

DREAM INTERPRETATION THROUGH THE AGES

Dreams must have been around for millennia but were first recorded when early civilizations were at their height. We know little of prehistory—though there are beautiful cave paintings all over the world, still being discovered. Yet they have kept their secrets. We may never learn if the vividly colored animal murals were inspired by the artists' dreams or plans for tomorrow's hunt.

> **" THE EGYPTIANS PRODUCED THE FIRST EVER BOOK ON DREAMS. "**

The ancient Egyptians, however, did reveal their dreams because they had the motivation to do so and the skills to describe them. But they— like other ancient races before and after them—regarded dreams mainly as signposts for the quality of life in their outer world. They had yet to explore the life of the inner world. That was to come thousands of years later.

Early forms of dream interpretation

The Egyptians produced the first ever book on dreams. Made of papyrus and discovered in sandy ruins near the Nile, *The Egyptian Book of Dreams* was written nearly 3,000 years ago, yet with no reference to the hidden depths of the mind. The Greeks and Romans were big on omens and portents, too. Psychologists today would chuckle at the priests' checklist of symbols and interpretations. But we must remember that symbols were tailored to the times. Seers were employed to look for good or bad fortune ahead for their masters.

One thousand years before that, the Chinese were placing great store on dreams as well. But they viewed them more as a means to explore the vast world of spirit, not as a representation of their own destinies or spiritual development. Limited accounts trickling down through the centuries sound more philosophic in content: "Is the dreamer seeing a butterfly, or a sleeping butterfly seeing the dreamer?" They were hardly a guide to self-help.

Bad omens

Our ancient ancestors' recorded dreams were polarized in their narratives, delivered in simplistic terms—success or failure. For example, in *The Egyptian Book of Dreams*, red ink on papyrus denoted bad tidings: red being the color of bad omens then. The Hebrews thought along the same lines, also not yet ready for the subtleties of dreams as we know them today. Only the aboriginal cultures embraced the spiritual concept of oneness with the world, understanding that everything and everyone was imbued with spirit, an invisible energy that connected all.

Somehow, a split occurred in civilizations where spiritual power was ascribed to unseen gods ruling from afar and making decisions for the people. Gone was the prehistoric sense of oneness with the universe, a joyous connection between the inner and outer world.

Its disappearance over the centuries was to cause catastrophic results, such as religious wars. That split from personal/divine power to divine monopoly was a serious loss, despite society's giant technological strides.

DREAMS AS DIVINE GUIDANCE

Our more recent ancient ancestors believed divine guidance came only from *without*. Biblical stories emphasize this, with constant reference to those celestial voices and visions dreamed by the prophets and reported to the multitudes. Yet ordinary people may have been able to foretell the future, with the more prudent dreamers keeping quiet—either unable to record their prophecies or, more likely, remaining silent through fear of reprisal.

Dangerous times

If a dream held a message or glimpses of the future not foretold by an accepted prophet of God, it was blasphemous to early Christians. They had embraced the monotheistic 18th-dynasty Pharaoh Akhenaten's insistence that there was only one God (as did Moses, who was raised in Egypt), communicating His wishes through a chosen few—chiefly His main followers. Joseph and Daniel are recorded to have received dozens of dreams from God, faithfully reported in the Bible.

But ordinary people kept silent—for the next 1,000 years or so. Then two Europeans in the 15th and the 16th century began taking risks, despite the fear of punishment. One such was Old Mother Shipton of Yorkshire, England, who described her visions in rhymed couplets, largely domestic in content—though she did predict horseless carriages, which came hundreds of years later, and that iron boats would navigate the seas. (She also predicted

the world would end, 211 years before the Mayans' inaccurate forecast for this century, so her gift was at times flawed.)

Burning witches for presumed rejection of the Church's teaching started in southern France in the 14th century. That grim practice spread to England in the 16th century. Mother Shipton avoided a terrible death by disguising her dream visions in verse: hard to decode clearly enough to condemn her to the fires.

A fellow sensitive, French-born Nostradamus penned *Les Propheties*, a set of extraordinary insights (did he dream them, or use a crystal ball?) in dense quatrains published in 1555. The book became a bestseller over the next few centuries and, incredibly, is still in print.

Many researchers since have been skeptical of his prophecies, yet the Provençal physician is credited with forecasting the two World Wars, nuclear destruction, the attack on the World Trade Center, and catastrophic climate change.

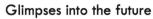

PRECOGNITIVE DREAMS

By the 19th century, recognition of the value of the inner world had arrived. Sigmund Freud pioneered this, realizing his patients were struggling with far deeper problems not recognized by the conscious mind. The mystery of precognitive dreams coming from the same realms had yet to be revealed until his colleague, Carl Jung, conceived his theory of the collective unconscious—the concept that we are all connected with all things.

Glimpses into the future

It is widely believed that nearly half the population of the world has clairvoyant dreams—not of the dramatic kind listed on the next page, but day-to-day glimpses into the future. They can be tantalizing snippets or bewilderingly accurate pictures. Relevant to every single one is that they are always ahead of time.

It is public knowledge that governments worldwide have used people gifted with ESP to view remotely—an ability to acquire information about a distant place—for military purposes. So we might reasonably ask the question: Is there really any difference between officially accepted remote viewing (as it is called) and clairvoyant dreaming?

Quantum physics

Now quantum physics has paved the way to understanding the impossible. It is pointing to the likelihood that precognitive material is a valid phenomenon, for time—as we've known it—now appears meaningless at the subatomic

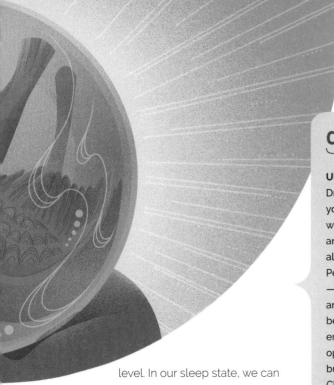

level. In our sleep state, we can trace old friends on the other side of the world, have a chat, embrace, and be back home for breakfast.

Clairvoyant dreamers

Clairvoyants—men and women with extra sensory perception (ESP)—and precognitive dreamers all seem to have one thing in common: somehow, they tap into a timeless zone where the past, present, and future are one. Here are just a few examples:

» Abraham Lincoln dreamed of his death just before his assassination.

» Albert Einstein's theory of relativity came to him in a dream.

» Beatles musician Paul McCartney composed "Yesterday" after hearing the melody in a dream.

» Golfer Jack Nicklaus dreamed of a new way to hold his golf club for victory.

» Novelist Robert Louis Stevenson first saw Dr. Jekyll and Mr. Hyde in a dream before writing his famous book.

CASE STUDY: REBECCA

UK research scientist and television presenter Dr. Christopher Evans once told Rebecca: "If you can bring proof of a clairvoyant dream, I will believe you." Hearing the mail carrier arrive a few weeks later in December, she alerted her husband: "I've just dreamed Peggie has sent an airmail from the States —something to do with an Egyptian mummy and clothing in blue-green. Please note this before I go downstairs and open the envelope, if it's there." He did. She then opened Peggie's letter, which asked her to buy a robe in blue-green for "Mummy's Christmas present." Rebecca called Dr. Evans and arranged to meet, but he politely refused to accept the sequence of her story. He insisted that she'd already read the letter, imagining later that she'd dreamed the letter contents before she opened it.

So most scientists continue to hold their stance, while psychics hold theirs—a deadlock between the two, it seems. But there is hope. As eminent American cell biologist Dr. Bruce Lipton says in his best-selling book *The Biology of Belief*: "I truly believe that only when Spirit and Science are reunited will we be afforded the means to create a better world."

DREAM SKILLS

GROUNDWORK FOR DREAM RECALL

Therapy has become increasingly holistic, and the body, with its nonverbal knowledge, is recognized as an important area for self-awareness. Through observing and checking in with the body, you can learn a great deal. Muscular tension, trembling, hot or cold sensations, and so on are indicative signs of emotions you have experienced. Practice the skill of tuning in to these to help dream recall.

Tune in to your body

As memories drift through your mind after a recent dream, your body will also have been involved as the dream unfolded. For instance, it may have been reliving making love to a former partner. Not always discernible but in reality fully present, that body is remembering.

Fear—our primal response to survival—is likely to top the list. Though actual survival is less of an issue in the developed world, psychological survival certainly is. Recalling unpleasant encounters and wanting to run away from them is experienced simultaneously by the dreamer's body. As countless bodywork researchers have discovered, memories are stored at a cellular level and will respond on cue if triggered by a dream narrative. Sometimes that body echo is obvious—but not always.

Focusing

American philosopher and psychologist Eugene Gendlin evolved a method to plumb those trapped somatic memories. He called his insight

> "DAILY MEDITATION WILL HELP YOU TO WORK MORE DEEPLY ON YOUR INNER WORLD."

Focusing; a process by which you contact hidden files of sensation. Calling it a "special kind of internal bodily awareness", Gendlin insists this is not an emotion—rather, it is a felt sense that can become meaningful only once you have worked your way inward to discover its significance.

Tense musculature can be the result of suppressing hurt or angry feelings in childhood. A young child does not yet have the brain development to challenge and deal with shock, however innocent; Focusing may help to release you from its grip. You can do this on your own, following Gendlin's six suggested movements (see Further Reading on page 211). Failing this, find a qualified body therapist trained specifically to work with somatic issues.

Mindfulness

Mindfulness is another valuable skill, in which you train yourself to notice consciously what you are thinking and feeling while it happens, here and now. For this, we largely use the right side of our brain, the seat of intuition and imagination. Meanwhile, the left side deals with logic, penetrating the outside world. When these two sides are in balance, all is well. Too often, the left hemisphere is overworked—consider business, politics, and law—and though essential, the resulting overthinking can blur what the psyche is trying to convey.

So you may find it hard to start with. Seek out a quiet space to sit and focus on the sound of your breathing. Try gently accepting your thoughts as they arise, then simply spiral back to the sound of your breath to quiet a chattering mind and prepare an inner space for creative thought. As psychotherapist Nigel Wellings, author of *Why Can't I Meditate?*, says, "By being mindful, we can catch our self in the moment going along well-worn tracks we now know do not serve us well and consciously choose to do something different."

Daily meditation will help you work more deeply on your inner world. As well as helping to transition to a more open mindset, it also reduces stress levels—this is science-backed—calms the mind, and can prepare you for a deeper quality of sleep for your dreaming life.

TIPS FOR DREAM RECALL

Always keep a notebook and pen by your bedside. The dream sequence too easily fades the moment day-to-day thoughts fill your conscious mind, such as "It's time to get up and get moving." The crucial aspects may be lost forever if you fail to scribble those waking memories down at once. Some people make themselves turn on the light in the middle of the night if a powerful dream impacts them sufficiently and they know they should note it or lose it.

Write notes

The moment you surface to consciousness, aware you have just come out of an important dream, grab your notebook and fill the pages with every detail you can capture. (See pages 37–39 for guidance on the kind of things you should be writing down here.) Try not to make it short and factual: this is not a business meeting between conscious and unconscious. Key qualities of the dream message may hide in the less obvious.

If it proves impossible to get anything written—mornings are full of domestic activity and other outer-world demands—then try to memorize at least one word (for example, "cars") and keep it in mind until you can record the rest. You are bound to lose out on the full record, but this encourages you to practice dream journaling and will at least help you get started.

Keep a dream diary

Keeping a dream diary is not only an interesting record of your life, but also allows you to look

> " REMEMBER, YOUR DREAMING SELF KNOWS A HUGE AMOUNT MORE THAN YOUR WAKING SELF DOES. "

back on your past emotional states. You may be amazed at the insights your diary offers. Even on a week-by-week or monthly basis, reading through your written words at the height of the dreams' impression will prove intriguing, if not revealing. It is not always possible to decode a dream on the same day. Events may need to unfold for the full significance to be understood. (See pages 36–41 for step-by-step advice on how to decode your dream.) Remember, your dreaming self knows a huge amount more than your waking self does: allow it to have awareness of coming activities or encounters, even if this would not be called a precognitive dream. (See pages 28–29 for more on precognitive dreams.)

Analyze your felt sense

Once you have written the dream story down, make sure your felt sense—as described by psychologist Dr. Eugene Gendlin in his book *Focusing* (see Further Reading on page 211)—has also been noted. By felt sense, we mean to check out how the body is feeling—what tensions or otherwise have been generated by the dream. (See page 32 for more on this method of insight.) Your bodily sensations can provide vital memory triggers.

USEFUL TOOLS

A hardback notebook
Keep a little notebook—preferably unlined, because you might want to make a quick sketch to illustrate the narrative—by your bedside. Flimsy, loose pages are not a good idea, as they are little better than the back of an envelope—plus they get lost.

A journal
Dream journals are to be taken seriously. They hold precious records from your unconscious self trying to help you consciously grow and move forward.

A small flashlight
It is sensible to have a small flashlight nearby, especially if you are concerned about not waking up a partner. Smartphone flashlights are not recommended because they cast a strong light—as would, of course, a bedside lamp.

A smartphone or voice recorder
Speaking your thoughts into a smartphone or other recording device is good, but disturbing another might be an issue unless you tiptoe to the bathroom.

35

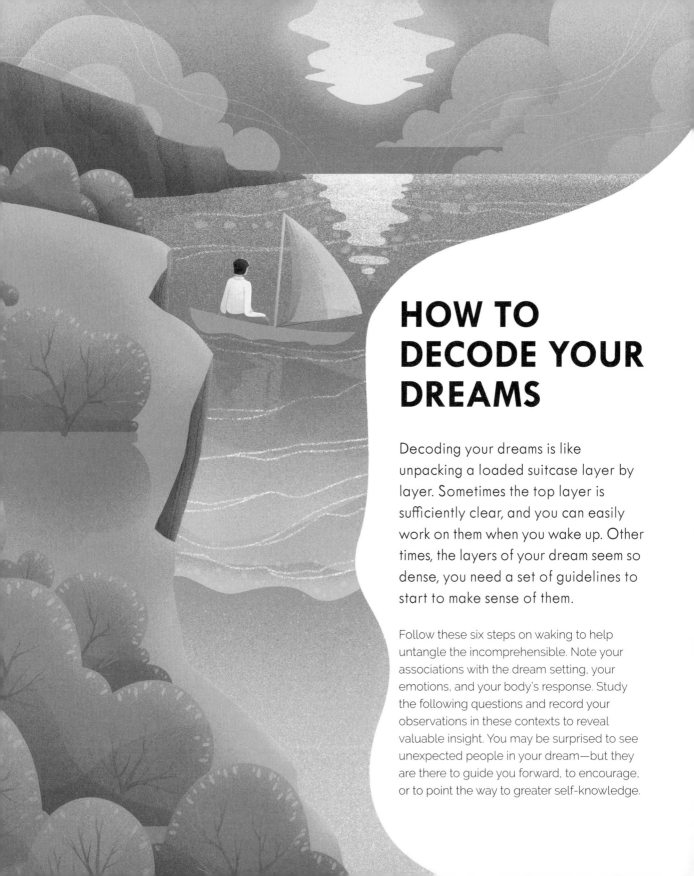

HOW TO DECODE YOUR DREAMS

Decoding your dreams is like unpacking a loaded suitcase layer by layer. Sometimes the top layer is sufficiently clear, and you can easily work on them when you wake up. Other times, the layers of your dream seem so dense, you need a set of guidelines to start to make sense of them.

Follow these six steps on waking to help untangle the incomprehensible. Note your associations with the dream setting, your emotions, and your body's response. Study the following questions and record your observations in these contexts to reveal valuable insight. You may be surprised to see unexpected people in your dream—but they are there to guide you forward, to encourage, or to point the way to greater self-knowledge.

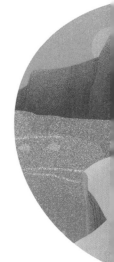

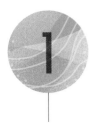

WHERE ARE YOU?

≫ **What is the setting of the dream?** Is it sunny and bright or in darkness? Is it outdoors or inside? Upstairs or in the basement?

≫ **Does the setting remind you of anyplace familiar to you?** Is it reminiscent of somewhere you spend time in waking life, or does it reflect a place from your childhood or more recent past?

≫ **What association does this dream location have for you?** Does it give rise to happy or uneasy feelings? At first, feelings may have been of one kind, then changed to others as the narrative unfolded. These feelings are an essential backdrop to the images—an important part of the puzzle.

WHO IS IN THE DREAM?

≫ **Are you alone, with another, or with a group of people?** Are they well known to you? If not, do they remind you of someone (however vaguely)? In dream interpretation, it is a person's perceived qualities that matter, not their appearance. Perhaps, alternatively, they are blank-faced strangers?

≫ **How do you feel when you can identify a person?** Friend or lover? A famous character? Write down in your dream journal what comes up in your mind as you reflect upon them.

≫ **When or how did this person or these people make the most impact on you in waking life?** This might be a clue to their unexpected appearance now.

≫ **Who is the chief person in the dream?** According to Carl Jung's theory, this man or woman can be a part of yourself, symbolizing your masculine (*animus*) or feminine (*anima*) energies. Alternatively, he or she could be representing one of your characteristics (though it may be disguised) or playing out a part of you largely disowned in waking life. We all have subpersonalities tucked inside our unconscious world.

Continued ≫

HOW DO YOU FEEL?

>> **Does the immediate waking feeling bring instant happy recollection of some past experience?** You might even feel like weeping as you realize a familiar figure in your dream, so wonderful to "see" again, does not now exist in the outer world—maybe a partner, a parent, or a loved one.

>> **What emotion does a strong memory of your dream call up?** Is it warm affection, embarrassment, loathing, or fear (these are examples only)?

>> **How did you feel in the dream?** Your feelings within the dream narrative will tell you the truth, the raw reality of your own authentic feelings about which you may not have been fully aware. Perhaps you try to hide (even from yourself) timidity, shyness, a lack of confidence, or a reluctance to confront in day-to-day life. But these secrets are well known to your psyche, anxious at this point to bring those emotions to the surface to be faced and dealt with.

HOW DOES YOUR BODY FEEL?

» **While you were dreaming, were physical sensations triggered in your body?** Sexual feelings may or may not be conveniently carried forward, but other bodily sensations are equally as important to observe.

» **Is your body tense following some distressing or frightening episode in your dream?** Try exaggerating that tension (you can do this while still lying down) to the point of physical discomfort. What comes up in your mind? Linked no doubt with the dream content, it may have brought more material to the surface from the depths of your unconscious: some trapped sensation, locked in at a cellular level.

» **Explore your felt senses.** What is the exaggerated pain in your rigid neck muscles recalling? Are your arms, buttocks, calves, and shoulders tensed, as if for action—hitting out, running away, or protecting yourself? These felt senses might prove to be vital clues in decoding the dream's message.

Continued »

WHAT EVENTS LED UP TO THE DREAM?

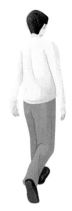

>> **What happened the day before the dream?** Often what happened during the course of the day is crucial—dreams often arrive that night, as if on cue, and their appearance now could more than likely prove to be a commentary on the day's thoughts or activities.

>> **What happened the week before?** The dream could be concerned with the overall picture of the preceding week, providing a subtle commentary on your day-to-day life.

>> **Have you recently had to make any major decisions, or have you been worried about trivial issues?** These can absorb waking energy and drain your emotional reserves. This is where helpful dreams come into their own: they point the way forward or show a new way to leave those anxieties behind.

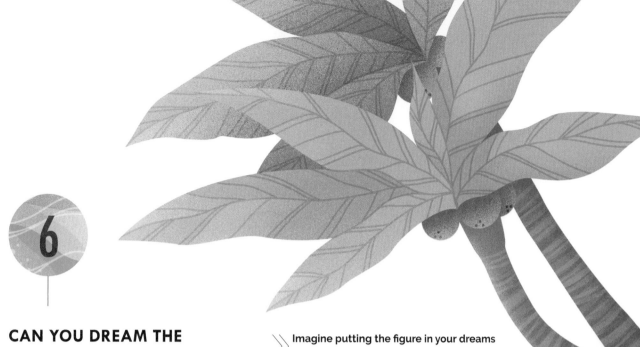

6

CAN YOU DREAM THE DREAM ON?

>> **If you follow some interesting opportunity in a dream scenario, what might happen now if you imagined going forward with it in real life?** Even if the narrative seemed to end conclusively before you woke up, try taking it further. This is not unlike meditation.

>> **Would you want to seize the chance offered, or definitely reject it? Why?** Notice your emotions as you ponder these choices: they could be helpful in resolving waking-life decisions. Try having an imaginary conversation with whoever seems relevant in the dream and see if you can formulate clearer perspectives. This method is called Active Imagination (as Carl Jung describes it), but many psychotherapists use similar means to reach a client's conscious awareness.

>> **Imagine putting the figure in your dreams (remember, it might be a part of yourself) literally into a chair.** Face that imagined figure and introduce a dialogue. Ask questions such as "Why are you so bored with your life?" or "You seem unhappy. Would you like to tell me about it?" Responses within your own head may come as a surprise, or even be illuminating. If the imagined figure in the chair across from you is indeed a hidden part of you, perhaps a critical or fearful subpersonality is longing to be acknowledged and integrated. Exploring that awareness at this point could yield some interesting insights into what is normally hidden from yourself.

Continued »

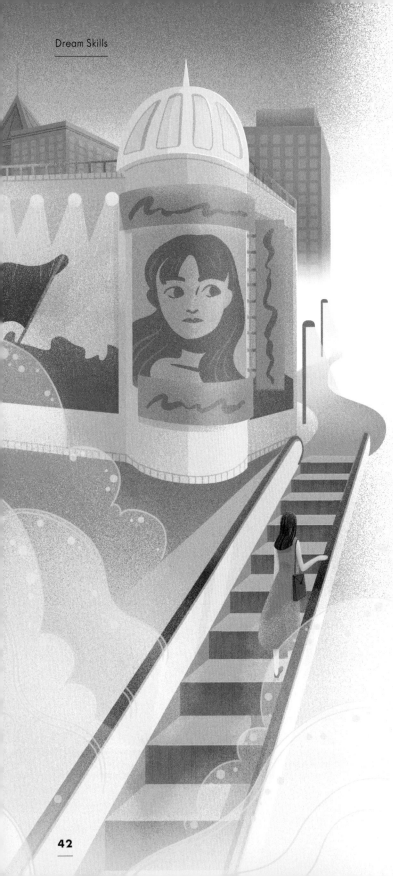

CASE STUDY: MARTHA

Martha was considering leaving her husband of 30 years. She struggled to find a solution to reconcile such a life-changing move. Here, we see a dream of Martha's and how, through decoding it using our six steps, she found in its message the motivation to move on.

THE DREAM

"I was at a summer festival, lying naked on the grass, though partially covered. A man came and lay beside me, putting a hand on my arm—not in a sexual way, rather in a manner that was soft and kind. Then the band played "Can't Find My Way Home" by Blind Faith. It felt significant to my personal dilemma. Next, I was upstairs in a restaurant where they sold expensive accessories. I liked a handbag and a wallet, then discovered I had left the restaurant still holding them: I'd forgotten to pay! Tomorrow, I'd go back, but somehow I didn't want to pay for the wallet.

Then an escalator I took away from the restaurant carried me like a train to a different part of town. It was unfamiliar, and once off the train, I noticed a theater. I don't like theaters—something about a stage performance fills me with dread.

An old woman appeared, walking briskly toward me in a businesslike, no-nonsense way, and I asked her for help in showing me the way home. She pointed firmly to a road I did not recognize. Somehow knowing she was right, I took it."

THE INTERPRETATION

WHERE ARE YOU?

The music festival is a familiar setting, as is a restaurant. These are places that are a part of Martha's everyday life. Then she finds herself heading out of town, out of her comfort zone. There's a theater here—a place that reminds Martha of how her dad took her to inappropriate places when she was little, where she felt awkward and ill at ease.

WHO IS IN THE DREAM?

A man lies beside Martha at the festival. He is her *animus*, her masculine self. Later, an old woman approaches her—the Wise Woman, in Jungian terms—and seems so certain of the way home. "Home" is not where she lives—it's her marriage, her faded relationship smothering her identity. She longs to take a new path, nurture her creativity, and find an authentic self.

HOW DO YOU FEEL?

Martha is enjoying the warmth of the sun at the festival. Once in the restaurant, when she sees the objects she has taken, she feels no guilt, but rather that the wallet holding her identity cards and personal details already belongs to her. It's her identity! As she finds herself traveling to an unknown part of town, she feels determined yet anxious. On waking, she feels as if a weight has been lifted from her at last.

HOW DOES YOUR BODY FEEL?

Martha's body tenses as she recalls the theater scene from the dream—the uncomfortable childhood emotions associated with the theater rising to the surface. She now realizes her husband John actually replicates those negative feelings.

WHAT EVENTS LED UP TO THE DREAM?

Martha and John had been having many arguments over recent months. She was growing increasingly weary of trying to make sense of his behavior and was torn between her grown-up children's reactions to her leaving him and her determination to get out of the marriage.

CAN YOU DREAM THE DREAM ON?

She wonders where that road leads and imagines herself traveling down it, aware of a growing sense of excitement as she walks into an art college. Martha sees herself teaching art—and loving her new life, in balance with her masculine and feminine self as never before.

"

DREAMS ARE OFTEN MORE
PROFOUND WHEN THEY
SEEM THE MOST CRAZY.

"

SIGMUND FREUD
THE INTERPRETATION OF DREAMS

LUCID DREAMING

Have you ever been aware that you are taking part and directing a dream and that you are stage-managing what happens next? This is called lucid dreaming, scientifically accepted as fact despite the strangeness of the concept. After all, how can anyone gain control over a normally "nonvolitional process," as sleep scientist Matthew Walker points out in his book *Why We Sleep?* Is functioning at two different levels really possible?

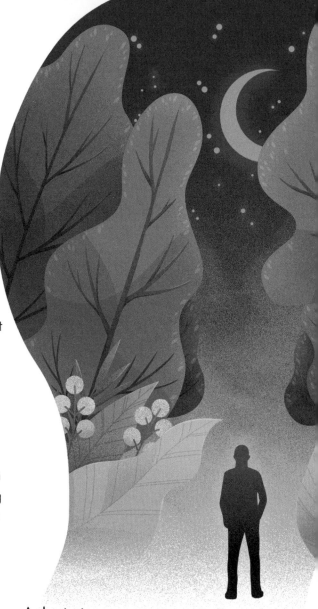

Walker describes how habitual lucid dreamers were taught in laboratory tests to give predefined eye movements to inform the researchers once they had gone to sleep. Three deliberate eye movements to the left, for example, showed the dreamer entering the lucid state and then (prearranged) two to the right, plus—incredibly—a clenched hand.

Fewer than 20 percent of the population can dream lucidly—these gifts are tantalizing potentials through which, perhaps, we may one day reach a more accessible connection between inner and outer worlds.

A shortcut

So what happens in lucid dreaming? Sometimes it is possible to see the person from whom you want an answer and then conduct a helpful conversation. It may be possible to shortcut the waking process of recording and decoding and learn about your dream while you sleep. If you are one of the lucky small percentage who often dream lucidly, then think of the creative possibilities open to you.

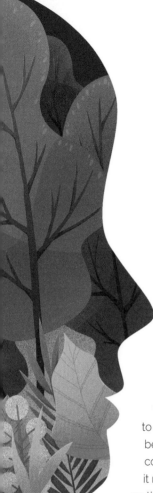

Learning to be lucid

You could experiment by imagining some everyday object in meditation, focusing on it several times daily. Tell yourself you will see it in your dreams and be able to touch it. Now you have begun the process to command lucid ability—but it needs dedication to keep up the practice.

Some people manage to teach themselves lucid dreaming by checking out during the night whether they are awake or dreaming, then commanding themselves to reenter the dream. Bizarre as it sounds, this "reality testing," as Stephen LaBerge of Stanford University and founder of The Lucidity Institute suggests, helps you move in and out of your dream world, recognizing from clues whether you're dreaming or awake. Ultimately, you might be lucky and become one of the hundreds of thousands of people who claim to be able to dream lucidly, potentially experiencing rarefied levels of mental activity and learning how to problem-solve during your sleep.

CASE STUDY: OWEN

A businessman whose health was deteriorating due to his obsessive drive dreamed he was talking to his younger self. A small boy, about 7 years old, was looking miserable. Owen, aware he was conducting a real meeting, felt anxious to help this sad little boy and knew he could direct what was happening. As they talked, he realized he was talking to a young version of himself, and—still in the dream—began to weep with sympathy to see this child's misery.

"What's the matter, why so sad?" he asked little Owen. Came the swift answer: "You've been too busy to have fun. You're miserable rushing about and so am I—please STOP!" And stop Owen did, requesting a sabbatical from work the next day. When he was ready to return, he stipulated easier schedules to give him more leisure time—and the fun that little Owen had insisted upon became a reality. Owen's health returned, and his career paradoxically became even more successful.

THE DREAM DIRECTORY

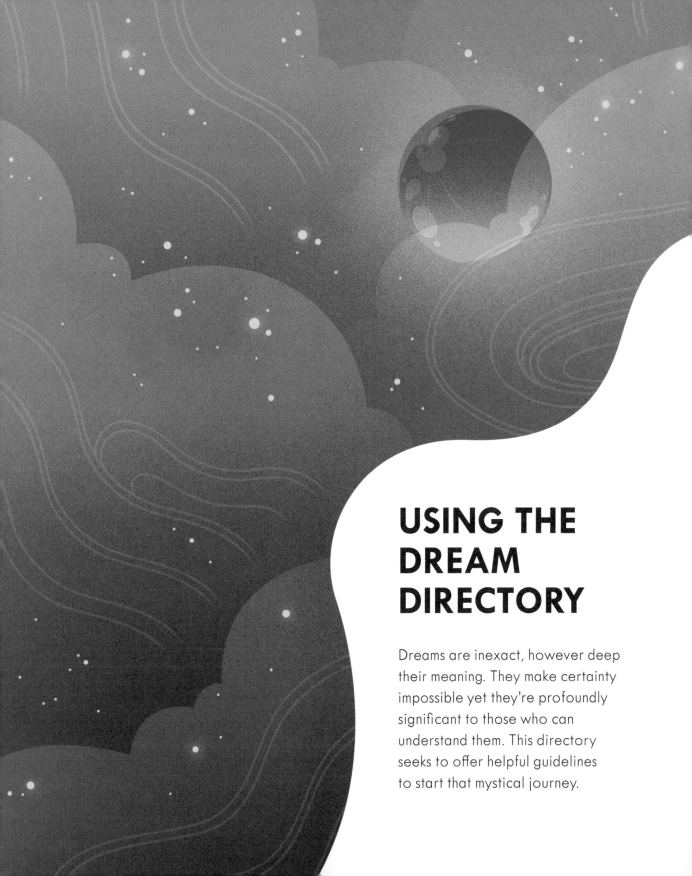

USING THE DREAM DIRECTORY

Dreams are inexact, however deep their meaning. They make certainty impossible yet they're profoundly significant to those who can understand them. This directory seeks to offer helpful guidelines to start that mystical journey.

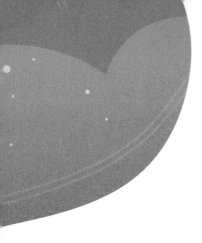

There was a time when readers opened how-to books and were confronted with their alarmingly simple format: "A black cat crossing your pathway brings good luck." More knowledge of psychology, the brain, learned behavior patterns, trauma, and even quantum physics has come forward in recent years to point the way to an infinitely wider backdrop to dreams.

Unlike the firm interpretative style of simple directories or results from internet searches, this directory sets out to provide different ways of looking at common dream scenarios. Included here are the most frequently occurring dreams most people recognize as theirs at some time or another. But there are also scenarios that are not quite so obvious that carry pertinent messages for the dreamer, showing just how subtle dreams can be. It also offers suggested action to take once the dream contents have been carefully worked through; this could validate what you're already doing, or instead could significantly steer you in another direction for a happier future.

Through understanding what sometimes appears as trivial dream content, we learn more about ourselves, why we do things, why we feel such and such—all through the insights offered by our psyche.

One size does not fit all

Before exploring the directory, a word of warning: self-help can be invaluable, but it is important not to fall into the "black cat means good luck" trap. Dreams are seldom simplistic and are always informed by our past history. You need to weigh all the material you can recall—as the decoding steps (see pages 36–43) and suggested actions to take throughout this chapter illustrate—or you might be getting the wrong slant on the dream.

For example, take mermaids: surely any woman would be enchanted by an ethereal vision of a mermaid? Not if the dreamer had experienced a miscarriage and now holds a horror of her fertility. A mermaid has no vagina, so there is no future danger of a lost pregnancy. A woman might not yet realize the connection, but decoding her dream could help her come to terms with her reality.

So before you reach any decisions about your compelling dream, remember that the canvas is broad: an anomalous appearance of something—or someone—in a simple scenario must be there for a reason. What memories, feelings, and connections come up as you reflect on them? They could hold the key to the answer you're looking for—and deserve to find.

AN OLD MAN OR WOMAN

Age equates with knowledge and wisdom. It can also mean slowing down and leaving running the world to the younger generation. The elderly have much to offer—and when they appear in dreams, those gifts are often profoundly important and not to be taken lightly.

THEY LOOK KIND AND EXPERIENCED

The kind and wise-looking old person appears to be pointing the way forward for you. He or she could be your archetypal wise self – if male, he's a senex or sage, like a wizard; if female, she's your wise old woman crone. Either one has appeared to guide you in some way.

Action Quiz yourself on what's going on in your life that deserves some helpful guidance. Are you contemplating a change of some sort? Is it risky? Are you in need of a gentle nudge to drop that idea or to get on with it?

THEY ARE CARRYING A CANE

An old person is carrying a cane. They appear frail, and their progress is slow. This could be a metaphor for being unable to move easily through your current situation.

Action Decide to examine your life from the viewpoint of it disabling you—maybe emotionally, intellectually, or even physically. (The latter could mean exhaustion.) Are you overworked? Playing too hard? Take heed of the metaphor. Are you meant to slow down?

THEY HAVE LINES ON THEIR FACE

Lines represent not only being a pensionable age, but can also show psychological exposure to life from prolonged stressful activity. Their presence could be acknowledging a hard life. If circumstances have meant suffering, the dream is a salute to your difficult journey of experience.

Action Unless you can identify that this face has been weathered by natural causes, your dream could be there to comfort you on life's tumultuous travels. If there's a way ahead to alleviate some of that stress, then act on it.

THEY **REMIND YOU OF A RELATIVE**

Unexpected old relatives appear in dreams. They might be a parent, grandparent, or elderly aunt or uncle, and they are present in some typical or unusual scenario, reminding you of the quality that most sums them up.

Action Consider those qualities: good or not so good? Your psyche may be running a script to point out how you need to change your behavior or attitude toward others. Remember, these old people carry your genes. How might you emulate their good qualities or work on improving the bad ones?

YOU **ARE OLD**

A dream group of wizened old people welcome you into their midst as one of them. You're their equal, no longer young, but this doesn't worry you.

Action We are often not fully aware of our fears. Growing old could be one of them. Age carries with it many potentially frightening possibilities, with loss of all kinds. But you need to bear in mind there are also positive aspects to old age. Encourage yourself to embrace that upbeat outlook.

UNFAITHFUL PARTNER

Betrayal is never pleasant. In all relationships, the pain of being wronged—however unlikely—is a dread that lurks in the back of the minds of couples no matter how happy they are together. Betrayal, of course, may never happen. But no one can ever be absolutely sure.

YOU **WANT REVENGE**

Your partner is being unfaithful somehow—and you feel like stabbing them in the back. You are furious and want revenge. But maybe it's not punishment you're after: you are possibly being unfaithful to a part of yourself here, and it's highly likely to be your ego.

Action Realize you are deceiving yourself in some way—perhaps ignoring warning signs from friends and family. Decide to check on all areas of your life in which you might not be behaving truly authentically.

YOU **FEEL JEALOUS**

You see your partner with another and feel envious. What is it about that man or woman that most affects you? If it's their unattractive qualities, are you surprised your partner finds them exciting? This could be your shadow at work in the dream—the hidden parts you've relegated to the unconscious because you've disowned them.

Action
Embrace your shadow material—bring it into the light and reflect on how what you consider unattractive might be fine with your partner. But you need to own your fears and discuss them with your partner.

YOUR **TRUST HAS BEEN BETRAYED**

Your partner is somehow being unfaithful; they no longer seem trustworthy. The dream unsettles you, and its uncomfortable storyline is hard to take. You are appalled and frightened, in the grip of dread. When you wake up, you realize this was more like a nightmare, playing out your deepest fears that your partner might one day be unfaithful.

Action Accept that you carry these worries and, if reality shows no sign of betrayal in your relationship, keep your fears to yourself. Believe in your partner's trustworthiness. It's a gift you can give the partnership that will reinforce the stability you crave. Respect their integrity, too; it's to be valued, not challenged.

YOU **ARE THE UNFAITHFUL PARTNER**

You dream of an exciting meeting with a new lover. You enjoy the encounter; it's fun and sexually fulfilling. You wish it could go on and on, and regret waking up to daytime reality. This dreamy partner has extraordinary magnetism— you want more! The sex was the greatest, and perhaps your current relationship doesn't match it.

Action Acknowledge the dream was fun and be relieved it unfolded in another world. But take a look at your relationship—the one you've just been "unfaithful" to— and ask yourself what steps you might take to improve what you have in the here and now.

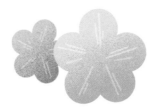

PREGNANCY

Pregnancy means fertility and a newcomer to the world. What must be acknowledged here is the fact that it is not always a joyous time—this baby might not be welcome. On the other hand, it could have been longed for after heartbreaking years of waiting. Either way, dreams featuring pregnancy can signify change.

YOU SEE A PREGNANT WOMAN

You are watching a pregnant woman walking toward you. Does her condition make you feel envy, or some other emotion? If you have had experience of being pregnant, or with a pregnant partner—good or bad—you might be reliving that time in this dream. But the question here is "Why have this dream now?"

Action Reflect on your feelings about seeing a pregnant woman in your dream. Have you processed them, regardless of being envious or relieved the pregnancy has nothing to do with you? If the sight of her pregnancy brings up many reflections, find someone with whom to discuss those thoughts.

YOU ARE PREGNANT

You are unexpectedly pregnant in your dream—and yes, a man can be, too—and feeling excited about the prospect of bringing new life into the world.

Action Being pregnant as a metaphor is all about creativity. This indicates new life in the widest sense. Take a hint and start creative moves in your life. Is there a book you've always meant to get started, or a project you want to develop? Pregnancy is all about gestation and delivery: be patient and wait for results.

YOU ARE THE BABY IN THE WOMB

Sometimes seeing or being a pregnant woman can be a sign you are about to give birth to a new part of yourself. This often happens when people are in therapy, but not necessarily so. That part of yourself is filled now with some potentially rewarding new being—perhaps one that makes you more assertive or confident, for example.

Action Plan how you would go about becoming more assertive or confident, or any other qualities you would love to possess. Trying ways to alter your normal pattern would be a creative move now, consciously following your unconscious lead that it's time to give birth to a new aspect of yourself previously hidden.

NO LONGER A VIRGIN

A pregnant woman by definition has lost her virginity. What can this suggest? If we take "virginity" as a metaphor here, we might be looking at a dream that indicates a loss of innocence. It could also be suggesting the dreamer needs to face the fact that adulthood requires behaving in a mature, wise way. Childhood self-indulgence is now in the past.

Action Decide what might be persisting to prevent you from psychologically growing up. Whether your actual virginity is an issue here or not, your psyche is indicating a need to reflect on what it means to be a mature woman or man.

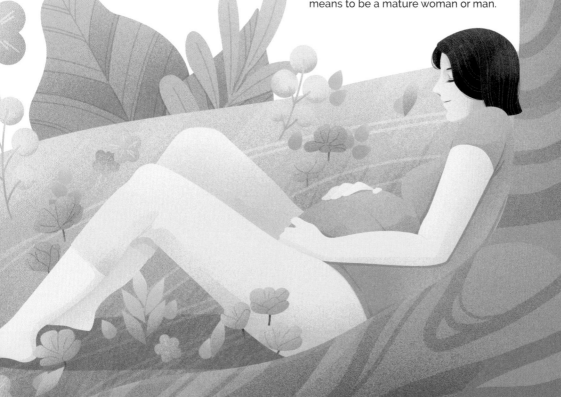

A FORMER LOVER

Nostalgia often drives this dream—a longing perhaps for a return to pleasures past. Do you want to find this lover again, or perhaps you are glad to be rid of that relationship? You've been reminded of the affair somehow. What's the message?

THE LOVER IS ELUSIVE

You are searching for a former lover, but you catch only glimpses of them. They are with a group of people or walking away from you. You call out or rush toward them, but you can never reach them.

Action Is your psyche warning you that the lover should not be called back to you? You could try to stop asking for a dream reunion. This might be a meeting with no solid future. If that lover intends to find you, wait for signs of their return.

YOU ARE WAVING GOODBYE

Themes of waving farewell may indicate you've said goodbye before the affair had run its proper course. Feelings of remorse or unease can accompany the narrative—whatever the storyline—and may suggest you and your partner have suffered unnecessary pain.

Action If it's not too late, get back in touch and ask to talk things through. Misunderstandings might be ironed out, mutual hurt soothed, and you just may get back together again. Resolve, however, not to pursue this if their response is negative. They've moved on now.

YOU'RE **LOOKING FOR SOMEONE TO MAKE YOU FEEL WHOLE**

A woman, believing she's looking for a former lover, might be searching for her *animus*: her masculine half to make her inner being more whole. Has a forceful, penetrative part of your personality been suffocated behind too much nonlinear, feminine behavior? If the dreamer is a man, then this applies to your *anima*—hunting for a gentler, empathic side to redress the imbalance.

Action Ask yourself if this rings true—the search needs investigation to help you lead a fuller life. Balance in the psyche is very important.

YOU **ARE ANGRY**

You dream of being back in a former relationship that was abusive and gave you no sense of peace. You wake feeling angry. Even though the episode is long gone and you parted company years ago, unpleasant feelings persist.

Action Realize you were caught in a situation over which you had less control than you do now. Away from that abusive relationship, you are free to make better choices.

YOU **ARE WISTFUL IT'S OVER**

In your dream, you relive the ending of your relationship. You realize you have no way of getting back in touch with your former partner and are left feeling wistful and full of regret. This kind of dream speaks of lost opportunity.

Action This is your chance to reflect on the breakup. If it was a good experience you thoughtlessly ended, think about your behavior and resolve to examine your part in the end of it. Were you reckless or maybe selfish?

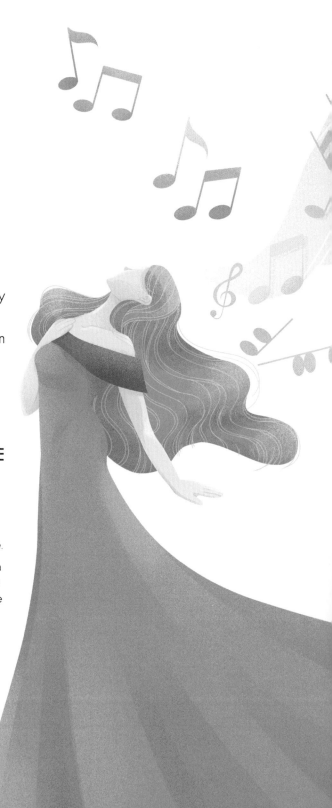

SOMEONE SINGING

Hearing a voice singing can bring comfort, joy, or amusement to the dreamer. Sometimes we can identify the singer, usually not so much a famous voice as someone familiar in our lives. The song may have significant lyrics or echo happy days from the past.

YOU RECOGNIZE THE VOICE

You dream of a familiar voice singing about how he or she feels about you—or how you would like them to feel! You may have put some wishful thinking into your unconscious mind, obligingly offering up a comforting tune.

Action Try capturing some of the words for a clearer meaning. Popular or classical pieces provide a cornucopia of loving phrases. Note the overall message and mention it to the singer, if you know them, and see where it goes from there.

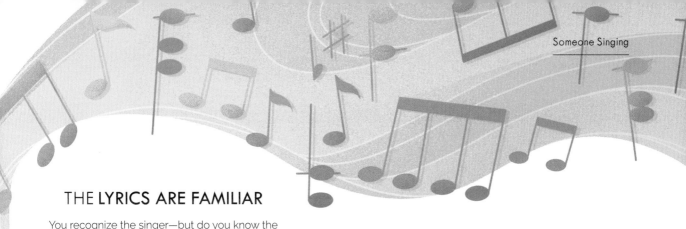

THE **LYRICS ARE FAMILIAR**

You recognize the singer—but do you know the words fully? What are your feelings when waking up with the melody still clearly in your head? It could surprise you with its unexpected statement or unequivocal hint about something your psyche needs to point out.

Action If you can identify the song, look up the lyrics on the Internet. You can learn a great deal from that search. Then consider what the sentiments mean: are they urging you to behave differently? Accept that your psyche found the best way to communicate by offering that particular song.

THE **COMMUNICATION IS** JOYFUL

You hear a joyful melody in your dream. It reminds you of the sound of love, and you recall earlier times when love flourished. This dream represents a joyful connection with your inner world.

Action If the singer is unknown, understand that the melody is a message of joy and potential. Think about how choral music at its best inspires: a spiritual gift, however unrecognizable, is being offered. Take it to heart.

THE **SINGING SOUNDS SAD**

You dream of hearing sad, mournful notes. Because this is about communication, the message could be reflecting a morose part of yourself. Have you been feeling down recently? Do you recognize someone else who is sad and the dream shows your sympathy?

Action Once you know who the sad one is here, move toward helping either yourself or your loved one. Acknowledging the pain or despair that is around can lead to some progress. Talk about it.

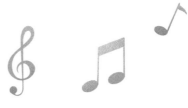

YOU **ARE THE SINGER**

You are singing your heart out in your dream. The voice you hear is your own, and the singer a creative, musical part of you. Have you not felt like singing lately? The dream is hinting at the need to heal that deficiency in your day-to-day life.

Action Accept that you've been low lately and the idea of singing for the sheer fun of it has seemed remote. Sing away or hum in the shower, or join a group who enjoys singing—it will lift your spirits.

KISSING A LOVED ONE

Kissing is an instinctual act, like a human version of the animal kingdom welcoming their precious newborn. It signifies bonding, affection, and connection. Dreams often reflect this reciprocal human trait—a primal need to be wanted and appreciated—and our longing for it to be mutual.

YOU ARE KISSING YOUR OWN IMAGINED CHILD

You dream of being an affectionate parent. But somehow you know there's no possibility of having a child of your own, and you realize you are mourning that fact by holding and kissing this small, soft being. The child looks just like you!

Action It could indeed be you—or rather, that little person you once were, still longing to be kissed and cuddled. Resolve to seek more affection from those nearest you. Be a loving parent to yourself; find comforting activities and plan outings with friends. Cuddle a cushion while pretending it's a young part of you. This can be a very comforting experience.

YOU ARE KISSING AN ANIMAL

A friendly, loving animal appears in a dream, and you feel a rush of affection. It seems to want to get to know you, reaching up for acknowledgment. You kiss its fur—it reminds you of childhood times, or just a furry toy animal you once treasured. You wake feeling relaxed and happy.

Action If life has been a bit tough recently, consider the charm of this dream. Your psyche has taken you back to earlier days, when contact with nature, animals, or playthings provided you with comforting continuity. Be grateful for the animal's appearance—it represents a part of what you loved. Now look for alternative ways to replicate those feelings. You need to treasure something in adulthood.

YOU **ARE BEING KISSED**

A dream with unpleasant sensations shows someone wanting to kiss you, declaring their love for you. You are being kissed by this person, and you feel powerless to stop it. Is this a replay of abuse in your childhood or a feared situation you dread ever happening to you or to someone you love?

Action If this was a replay, then remind yourself the abuse is in the past. If therapy is implied, take this dream as the prompt to seek help. It may be comparatively innocent: you simply don't like being kissed. If you otherwise like the loving one, explain your feelings and hope you're understood.

YOU **ARE KISSING AN OLD FLAME**

You dream of kissing an old flame in an unusual context. They walk up to you and kiss you on the brow—not the lips—and this is puzzling. Their behavior is not how you remember them when you were in love.

Action If the context has meaning for you, understand that your old flame is showing you a different kind of love now. What used to be a wildly erotic relationship has burned itself out, so enjoy the memories and accept that there's no going back.

> ## SO CAN DREAMS CHANGE SOMEONE'S LIFE? OF COURSE THEY CAN.

STANLEY KRIPPNER
DREAMS THAT CHANGE OUR LIVES

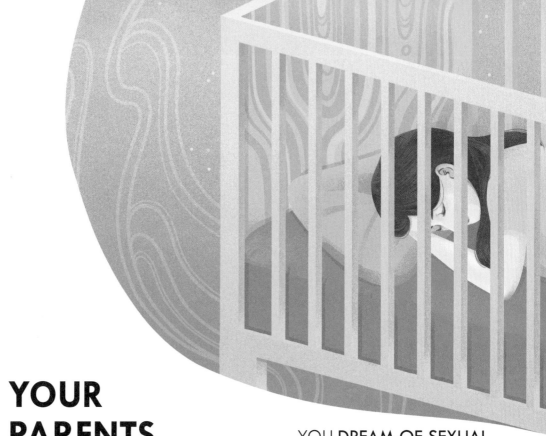

YOUR PARENTS

Anyone interested in the work of Sigmund Freud will know he regarded the Oedipus Complex as important—little boys must work through their need to kill off their father to marry their mother, and girls vice versa. Though outdated in part, Freud's theory persists: our dreams can be evidence of this. Another aspect of the relational bond—John Bowlby's Attachment Theory—also runs through our dreams to highlight how dependent we once were upon our parents' nearness to feel safe, or not.

YOU DREAM OF SEXUAL THRILLS WITH YOUR PARENT

Usually this dream occurs in young children who are unaware of sexual intercourse. However, their growing sense of connection—and bodily feelings—can induce sexually fired dreams. For adults, similar activity with the same excitement can be alarming to the dreamer. There is nothing to fear, however.

Action This dream is an echo of the Oedipus Complex. Take a look at yourself: are you missing a parent and longing for reconnection, but unsure how to get it? As a 4- to 7-year-old, you were likely to have experienced sexually charged dreams as the natural prelude to adult sexual activity. If your parents were unable to guide you through this phase by, for example, keeping firm bedroom boundaries while building your own growing sense of value, accept their mistake and move on.

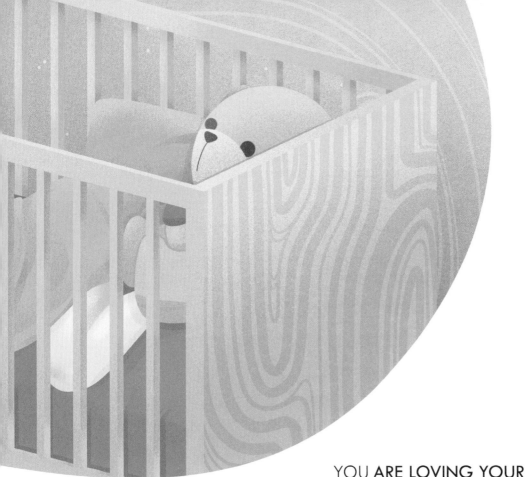

YOU ARE WANTING TO BE A CHILD AGAIN

You are with your parents in some family activity. It's a lot of fun and you are having the time of your life, laughing and joking with everyone. Your whole family seems so special—you are blissful in the dream.

Action Tell yourself it's fine to have this kind of dream: who wouldn't want that lovely dream? Being a grown-up can be hard work. Provided childhood held good memories, don't blame yourself for wanting to dip back into those times. Such a dream can refresh and support you as an emotional boost while you lead your adult life. But does that dream reoccur often? You may be yearning unhealthily for those days, so check out their frequency. Therapy might be needed.

YOU ARE LOVING YOUR PARENT'S AFFECTION

You are tucked in bed with a mild illness. Along comes your beloved parent with remedies—a hot-water bottle and all of your favorite magazines. You feel so safe and so wonderfully looked after that you hope they will make a decision to keep you with them until you get better—and long afterward. You love them so much, this is the perfect arrangement, and you don't want it to end.

Action This scenario shows you are still too attached to your mother or father—overly dependent. It's time you realized you must start separating from that reliance on your parent or parents. Psychological maturity is a long and painful path, but if you suspect you should, start taking steps toward autonomy. You will never lose the love you share.

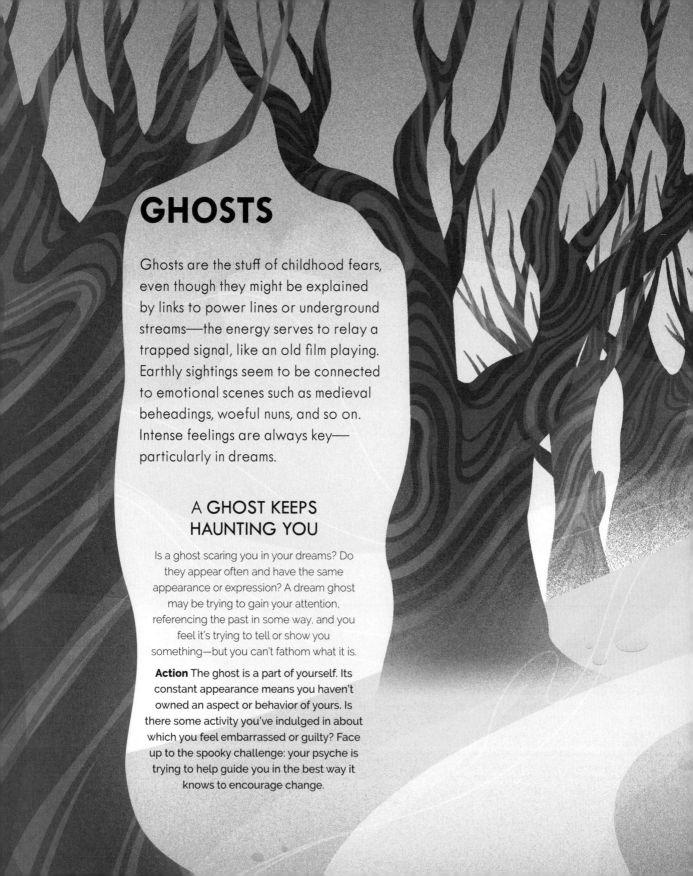

GHOSTS

Ghosts are the stuff of childhood fears, even though they might be explained by links to power lines or underground streams—the energy serves to relay a trapped signal, like an old film playing. Earthly sightings seem to be connected to emotional scenes such as medieval beheadings, woeful nuns, and so on. Intense feelings are always key— particularly in dreams.

A GHOST KEEPS HAUNTING YOU

Is a ghost scaring you in your dreams? Do they appear often and have the same appearance or expression? A dream ghost may be trying to gain your attention, referencing the past in some way, and you feel it's trying to tell or show you something—but you can't fathom what it is.

Action The ghost is a part of yourself. Its constant appearance means you haven't owned an aspect or behavior of yours. Is there some activity you've indulged in about which you feel embarrassed or guilty? Face up to the spooky challenge: your psyche is trying to help guide you in the best way it knows to encourage change.

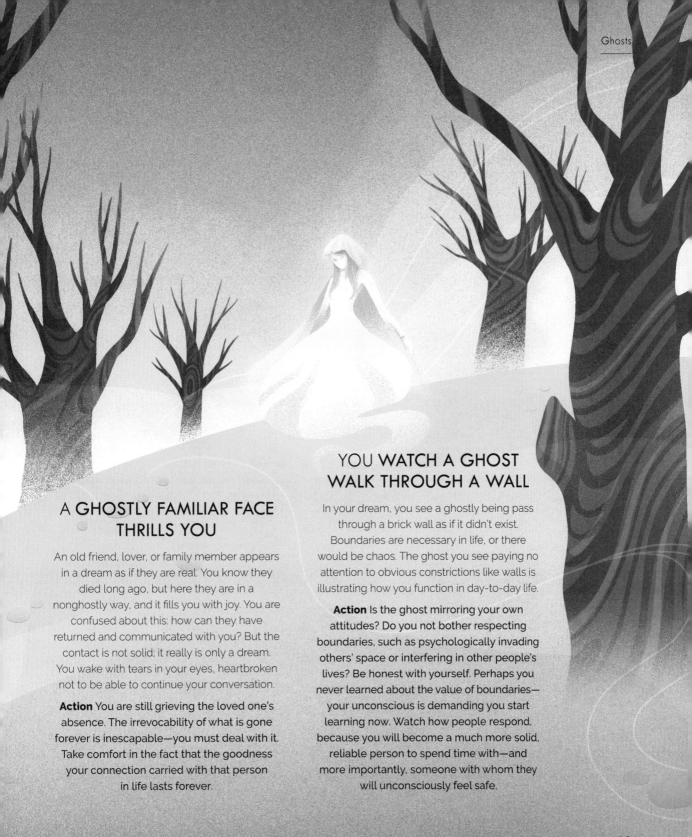

A GHOSTLY FAMILIAR FACE THRILLS YOU

An old friend, lover, or family member appears in a dream as if they are real. You know they died long ago, but here they are in a nonghostly way, and it fills you with joy. You are confused about this: how can they have returned and communicated with you? But the contact is not solid; it really is only a dream. You wake with tears in your eyes, heartbroken not to be able to continue your conversation.

Action You are still grieving the loved one's absence. The irrevocability of what is gone forever is inescapable—you must deal with it. Take comfort in the fact that the goodness your connection carried with that person in life lasts forever.

YOU WATCH A GHOST WALK THROUGH A WALL

In your dream, you see a ghostly being pass through a brick wall as if it didn't exist. Boundaries are necessary in life, or there would be chaos. The ghost you see paying no attention to obvious constrictions like walls is illustrating how you function in day-to-day life.

Action Is the ghost mirroring your own attitudes? Do you not bother respecting boundaries, such as psychologically invading others' space or interfering in other people's lives? Be honest with yourself. Perhaps you never learned about the value of boundaries—your unconscious is demanding you start learning now. Watch how people respond, because you will become a much more solid, reliable person to spend time with—and more importantly, someone with whom they will unconsciously feel safe.

DEAD BODIES

The idea of dead bodies may not be a comfortable one, but as we are born, so must we die. Death can be the beginning of new life, much as a newborn baby faces transformation from one state to another. Dreams, therefore, will often figure within this concept of change.

YOU SPOT A FAMILIAR DEAD BODY AMONG OTHER CASUALTIES

A battle has been waged and the scene is strewn with bloody victims. Dead bodies are everywhere and you have no idea who they are. Then suddenly, one body is clearly someone you recognize. It is that of your beloved partner or friend. What does this dream death mean to you?

Action Whether a precognitive metaphor for the death of a close connection with a particular person or your own sense that a relationship is doomed and coming to a natural conclusion, it certainly indicates the end. A dead person, once vital and rigorously alive, is no more. Accept the relationship death, mark the grave, and move on.

YOU ARE BURYING A CORPSE

Someone has died, and you find yourself digging a deep hole. There is a dead body to be buried, and you are responsible for hauling it into the muddy cavity and covering it with earth. It's an unpleasant, lonely task yet you set about it willingly, as if you somehow know this is the right thing to do.

Action In Jungian terms, burying the corpse has significance: it means your inner Hero— the part of your personality compelled to rush in to the rescue—has had his day. He's exhausted, and it is high time now to "kill him off" in order to lead a less driven life. Be grateful for your psyche's hint and learn to stop rescuing everyone.

CASE STUDY: ANNE

Months before her vicar husband was diagnosed with a motor neuron disease, Anne had a vivid dream: she watched him peel off a painted carapace, representing a normal clothed person. Underneath was his own lifeless body, which he draped over the back of a chair. It was without muscle, structureless. Anne recorded the dream but got nowhere in decoding it. After Isaac's diagnosis, he steadily lost control over his muscles. On the day of his death, she glimpsed him looking like the man in her dream.

She discovered a secret diary Isaac had written over the previous 30 years. Throughout, he described extramarital affairs, about which Anne knew nothing. He'd called himself psychologically "unmuscled," "weak," and "paralyzed."

Those revelations changed her life. Isaac had always made *her* feel to blame for their unhappiness. Incapable of an honest, loving relationship, he revealed a mental disorder never diagnosed.

Anne finally understood the cause of their suffering. The explicit imagery in that timely precognitive dream now helped her come to terms with her anger and grief.

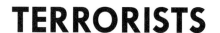

TERRORISTS

Terrorism is global, reported in our newspapers and on television every day. There is fear at pandemic level as angry men and women take to weaponry to mark their disgust or hatred. If we view the phenomenon as a metaphor, such brutality has its place in our inner world.

YOU **DREAM OF TERROR IN THE STREETS**

Terror fills your dream—there is panic everywhere, people screaming and running from danger. It seems gunmen are out to get them. Are you also a target? Where are you? Do you understand what motivates their fury?

Action Look at the dream as a metaphor and consider the terrorists' emotional drive. Decide what that might reflect in your life. If your boss, partner, or relative seems like a candidate for the gunmen, think of their perspective. Would a conversation be helpful with any of them, in which you express your own feelings?

YOU **ARE THE TERRORIST**

Killing people is wrong, and your conscious mind agrees—but unconsciously, the rule is different. You allow yourself a killing spree to rid yourself of wrongdoers against you. This kind of dream projects your unacceptable true feelings onto bad people so you can have the satisfaction of dealing with them.

Action Accept that you might want to point a gun at someone who annoys you. You secretly only want to terrify them, not kill. Terrorists, after all, are making a political statement where words no longer count. So consider using dialogue today: it can do no harm.

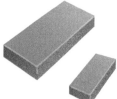

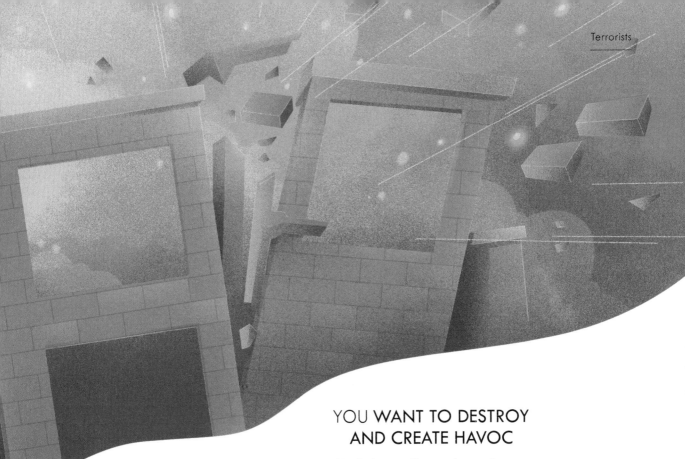

YOU **WANT TO DESTROY AND CREATE HAVOC**

You find yourself somewhere unknown, armed with weapons. All you can think of is destroying as much as you can see, creating havoc wherever you walk—like a terrorist. You do kill yet it gives you no satisfaction.

Action There is a part of yourself you want to destroy. You don't like what it is doing to you and others. Befriend that disliked part: perhaps it has been in the shadows too long and needs your help to adapt to the light.

YOU **SEE A VICTIM TURN INTO THE PERSECUTOR**

The dream shows a pathetic victim relentlessly hurt by the perpetrators in some way. Then as you watch, the victim gets out of their trapped state, runs away, and finds freedom. Perhaps a weapon is found, and that same person turns to face the persecutors. The roles are suddenly reversed!

Action Yes, this could be the dreamer caught in a dramatic triangle of victim turned persecutor. This is a wishful dream, living out your daytime plotting and scheming—but is it really the way forward? Consider the better route by upping your courage within the situation and, instead of being persecutor, turn mediator.

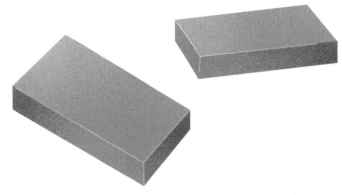

RESCUING PEOPLE

Being a hero—this is masculine, or *animus* territory—is often part of our psychological makeup. We play hero when heroism is not required. So there's a caveat here. Does it feed your ego and sense of self, needing to rescue in order to feel good?

YOU **RESCUE A CHILD**

Your dream shows kids in dangerous places taking risks. You see a particular child in danger. You hesitate, wondering if the parents might object, but you hurry forward anyway to carry that little child away from the perceived threat.

Action Your dreaming self did the right thing: perhaps this resonates with some episode in your own childhood. Now you are practicing taking charge of the situation, no longer helpless.

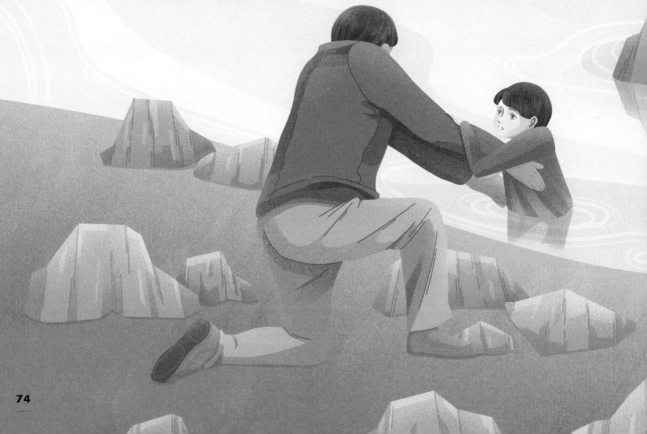

A FIRE THREATENS EVERYONE

Flames are endangering people, and you jump to the rescue. You feel it is your job to rescue them and imagine their gratitude when you pull them to safety. Fire engines arrive and firefighters get to work as you watch, feeling disappointed you are not also involved.

Action Realize how much importance you put on your need to rescue in any given situation, even when it may not be appropriate. Let others carry the load instead sometimes.

YOUR **HOME IS ON FIRE**

Are you helpless as flames devour your home? No one is there to rescue you, and your old independence and fight seem to have gone. Piece by precious piece burns up, and you despair about ever creating a comfortable living space again.

Action You are the house on fire—you may be suffering from burnout, needing to rest and recuperate. It is not always possible to rescue situations or people, and your exhausted psyche is showing you should stop. Take a vacation if you can and pamper yourself. Or try limiting the hours you work.

A **KNIGHT GALLOPS TO THE RESCUE**

Corny, but this familiar storybook rescuer often appears in dreams when you're looking outside for help. Instead of resolving your own difficulties, you give yourself a wishful scenario in which the archetypal hero arrives on his white horse and saves you.

Action Be your own brave knight! No need to find a white horse—just come to grips with the problem and discuss it with the right person. Solutions are there once you appreciate what your psyche is cleverly pointing out.

FEELING RESPONSIBLE FOR OTHERS

It can be a heavy burden to take on responsibility for other people, but often the burden does not need to be so weighty. Feeling responsible is different from *being* responsible: you have a choice over the first, even if you don't over the second. Dreams can be helpful in making you realize this.

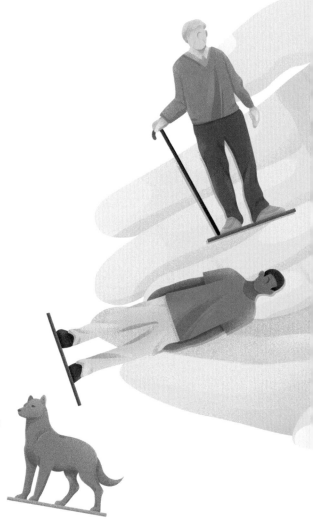

YOU FEEL YOU HAVE A DUTY TO PROVIDE CARE

You are excessively worried and concerned about a person or other people. You can't cope with the demands you *must* meet—otherwise, what dreadful outcome might there be?

Action This dream is about self-imposed duty. You might unconsciously be seeking self-importance in your life. Do you rush in to take over "to help people," when perhaps you are infantilizing them? Have you considered those people could do perfectly well without your intervention?

YOU ARE ACTING IRRESPONSIBLY

In your dream, pets need feeding and elderly parents need attention. You've neglected your responsibilities, and there's hunger and grief all around. You are full of remorse and wake up feeling miserable.

Action Resolve not to be careless in your duties, however full your day is. Delegate if necessary—be responsible about that, too.

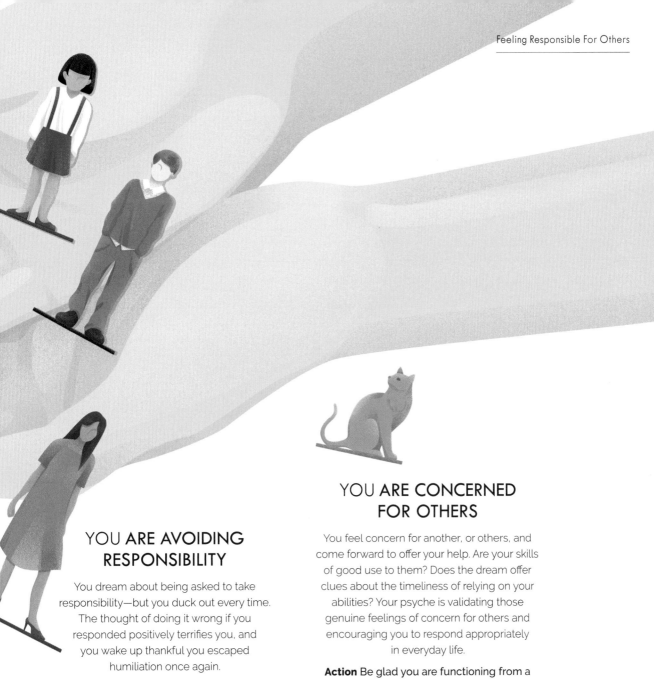

YOU ARE CONCERNED FOR OTHERS

You feel concern for another, or others, and come forward to offer your help. Are your skills of good use to them? Does the dream offer clues about the timeliness of relying on your abilities? Your psyche is validating those genuine feelings of concern for others and encouraging you to respond appropriately in everyday life.

Action Be glad you are functioning from a balanced inner world: you are mature in your outlook, coming forward when needed and withholding when best to let others look after themselves. It is more spiritually valuable to relinquish responsibility sometimes. Responsibility comes in various guises: know when to take it.

YOU ARE AVOIDING RESPONSIBILITY

You dream about being asked to take responsibility—but you duck out every time. The thought of doing it wrong if you responded positively terrifies you, and you wake up thankful you escaped humiliation once again.

Action Worrying about doing it wrong if you take appropriate responsibility has left you morally bankrupt. It's important to wake up to the fact you won't always get everything wrong. Those fears probably started in childhood with insensitive parents. Start taking responsibility, one step at a time.

STRANGER CARRYING A LONG OBJECT

There's usually something sexual about this kind of dream. Long objects are regarded as phallic and—unless there's definite contradiction to this theory in the context—we could assume the person carrying the object in your dream is connected in some way to eroticism.

THE **LONG OBJECT IS A BATON**

Surprisingly, this often features in dreams. After all, what is a conductor's baton for but to hold musicians together, making music? Can you see the parallel in your own life? What are you—or someone close—trying to conduct without too much intimacy being involved? A baton could represent distancing yet being fully in charge. Consider it, too, as a metaphor for a penis.

Action Sexual activity can be a wonderful, lively performance or a controlled, disconnected one. Think about your own—or your partner's—and decide to make changes if real connection and intimacy are missing.

THE **STRANGER IS CARRYING A SWORD**

A sword is a penetrative sign of masculine potency. If your dream stranger comes toward you brandishing his weapon, you may cower at the unknown ahead or enjoy the possibility of unbridled lovemaking. Either way, this might be a timely dream, but be faithful to its emotional content, too.

Action Ask yourself, why now? Is sex with a stranger an appealing idea? Or is that stranger your familiar sexual partner yet behaving in unexpected ways that you like—or don't like? Tell them about your dream and discuss openly what it might mean.

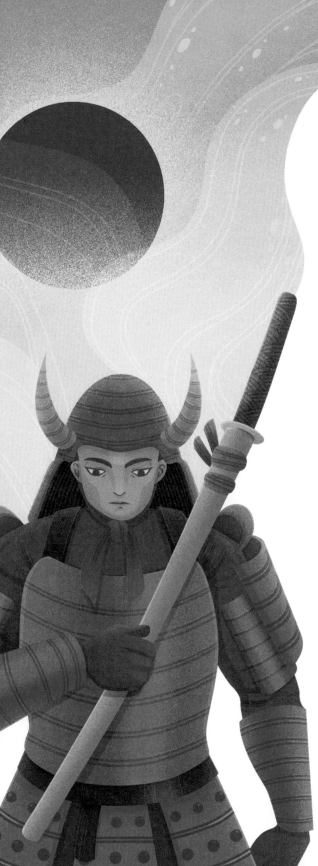

THE **LONG OBJECT IS PLACED AS A BRIDGE**

Any long object placed like a bridge could represent a penis. Here, it can be interpreted as bridging the division between the masculine and feminine self. That bridge, symbolic of the penis, penetrates and co-creates. This is a positive dream of encouragement despite its unlikely narrative.

Action Be glad your psyche has shown you in this graphic way a subtle hint about balance. You need to enhance whichever side is underdeveloped in your inner world. Because it is a masculine symbol bridging the gap in this dream, maybe you need to assert yourself more in life? Be more linear in your thinking, or more penetrating?

THE **PERSON WANTS YOU TO TOUCH A LONG OBJECT**

There's a room full of long objects of every description, and you get the feeling they are bad and have no right to be there. Someone picks one up and holds it out to you, eager for you to examine it. They seem overly concerned about your reluctance to reach out and touch. Fearful, you want to run away—but there's no exit to this room.

Action Are you afraid of sexual activity? Was there perhaps an inappropriate time in your history (childhood abuse often lies behind such fear) that still haunts you? Examine your attitude to current sexual encounters. If you suspect they have been influenced by that time, understand you have nothing to fear now. You are in control—there is a way out.

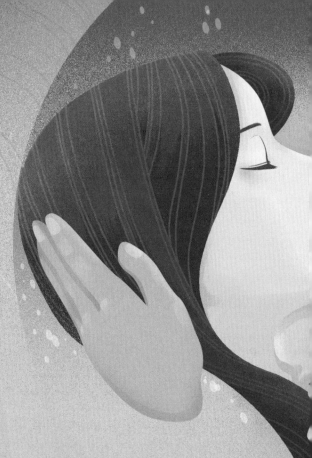

MAKING LOVE

Making love with a sexually fulfilling partner is one of the great pleasures of being human. Our bodies, mind, and spirit should all be involved in the best kind of physical joy; however, it is not always experienced by those who engage in sexual intercourse. Our dreams can reflect that joy— or deficiency.

MAKING LOVE WITH AN EX-PARTNER

You meet your ex-partner or lover at a gathering and find yourselves talking. Old memories come flooding back as you laugh about the good times, forgetting the bad ones. You make love. But it doesn't work and you wake up sad all over again, remembering why the relationship ended.

Action It is time to move on. You had unconsciously longed to reconnect because you believed the partnership brought all the qualities needed to make you feel fully yourself. But the dream showed clearly an end was inevitable. The shock needed healing. This is now the starting point to find a new love.

UNSATISFYING SEX WITH YOUR CURRENT PARTNER

Yet again, your partner has left you unfulfilled and angry after trying to make love. The dream setting is gray and colorless, the covers barely ruffled, and you climb out of bed and walk away. Your partner calls something out to you, which—though muffled—sounds as if they, too, are in distress.

Action Reflect on your own part in the difficulties. Unless there is a physiological reason for an inability to have sex, then maybe shyness, a lack of confidence, embarrassment, or any and all can apply to an unfulfilling time. It is up to you to determine who needs encouragement and how that might be achieved. Most importantly, sit down and talk about it.

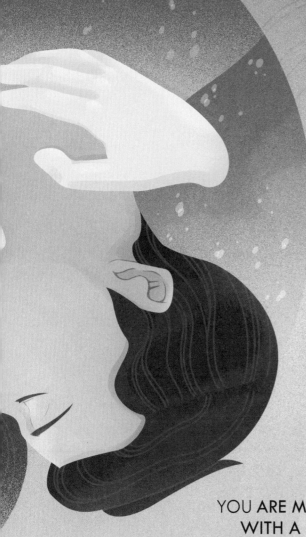

PASSIONATE SEX WITH A FANTASY LOVER

You are alone in a quiet area and see a powerfully attractive stranger. An instant rapport springs up between the two of you, and to your amazement, you are next making glorious, sensual love. You've never known such passion and are amazed at the intensity of the encounter.

Action Your real-life partner may not look like fantasy fodder, but they are as capable as you of bringing more satisfaction into your lives. Reflect on why your psyche is offering this blissful dream meeting—is it a nudge to come down to earth and to understand it's possible here? Work on it!

YOU ARE MAKING LOVE WITH A CELEBRITY

A famous person has chosen you for their partner: you are enfolded in the arms of a celebrity—because you, too, are one. Do you see yourself as an equal, consorting with other famous people?

Action This is probably a wishful dream, one that reflects a longing for glamor and recognition. It's easy to have an inflated idea of your appeal, in an unconscious search to compensate for what you may be lacking in your daily life. Perhaps it's time to accept that longing for the unlikely will only bring you disappointment. Learn to be a star in your own group.

WATCHING SEXUAL ACTIVITY

These days, watching sexual activity on a screen is commonplace, even if not universally favored. There is an emotional distancing involved when people are not participating themselves: their zest for vicarious living has become preferable to an authentic relationship, and perhaps they're losing out.

YOU WATCH FRIENDS MAKING LOVE

You are watching a couple you know and like making love in the dream, and you feel a painful sense of isolation. A lonely outsider, you feel excluded from something precious that they have obviously found together.

Action Ask yourself what it is that's stopping you from having a fully satisfying sexual life of your own. Consider what you need to do to find a partner.

GROUP SEX IS IN FULL SWING

You are in a room where group sex is in full swing, with everyone enjoying the excitement. Men and women are moving from partner to partner, couples are joining up with other couples for a foursome, and you feel a sense of loneliness. You long to find someone with whom to share sexual pleasure, to join in, but realize in the dream you want only real connection, not a superficial fun time.

Action Your innate wisdom has shone through in this dream: follow the instinctual response you felt there and don't seek out activities that will only bring transitory fun. Your needs are deeper than this—understand you are being urged to find a more rewarding connection with another.

YOU ARE ONE STEP REMOVED FROM DANGER

The dream shows sexual activity going on and it's wildly over-the-top pornographic. You feel lucky not to be involved (too racy!) but glad to be witnessing it all. You enjoy being there and have no sense of shame. You resent the dream ending when you wake.

Action This is one step removed from you being engaged in sexual activity and is without involvement. You have enjoyed plenty of sexual thrills without really being present. This is the stuff of voyeurism. Realize you need to move on and become involved at least in some sexual activity. It doesn't have to be raucous.

YOU ARE A SHY OBSERVER

You're watching sexual activity on television. Does the dream excite you? Do you feel fear, shame, or embarrassment? Was it a replay of a program you had watched in reality, maybe earlier that night? Did you feel involved in some way, or were you just watching? Note your reactions when you wake up and compare them with your felt sense.

Action Sexual feelings are easily stimulated, and a dream following a screen drama is normal. If the sexual scene came out of the blue, reflect on the feelings it has engendered: shame and embarrassment could suggest you are still shy about sex. Notice how your dream neatly placed you at a safe distance from the erotic action and determine to face those fears.

CHILDHOOD HOME

Dreams about childhood play an important part in our inner world. They remind us of the years when we had few responsibilities and enjoyed our freedom, or they serve to show how unhappy we were. Our home is where it all began—and dreams often place us there.

WISTFUL MEMORIES OF HAPPY TIMES

Your dream echoes happy times from when you were young. It shows scenes from childhood that remind you only of good, safe, and fun days with all your family and friends. This kind of recall can make you wistful for those uncomplicated years that you want to recreate in your current life.

Action Accept that those happy days belong to childhood and that you were lucky to have them. You cannot recreate such innocence again, however much you want to. If adult life needs a morale boost, invite yourself to an understanding friend's house and have fun with their young family.

YOU ARE WATCHING OTHER CHILDREN PLAYING OUTSIDE

You look out of the window and see children playing out in the sunshine. You long to join them, but there are responsibilities to look after someone indoors. Resigned, you turn sadly away from the window and go about your duties in the home.

Action You had to grow up too soon, through no fault of your own. You must accept the past; there's no going back. It's important to grieve for your lost opportunities, but be resolute in putting those memories behind you. Tell yourself you did your best. Now it's time to enjoy the present.

YOU ARE ROAMING FROM ROOM TO ROOM

You're moving from room to room trying to find something you need to take with you into your present life. You somehow sense that if you find that certain something, it will help lead you to your full potential.

Action Ask yourself why you have this need to look backward. What do you lack currently that has left a void that needs filling? Perhaps you missed out on learning something in childhood to help you reach your potential. If so, reflect on the deficiencies then and work out how to rectify them now where possible.

YOU ARE REVISITING YOUR CHILDHOOD HOME

As an adult, you find yourself looking at your old childhood home. With the magic stage management dreams can conjure, you see yourself as a child playing with siblings and friends. You are fascinated watching that interaction between you and the others. It seems important.

Action That interaction *is* important: the relational dynamic between you and them will tell you a great deal about who you are now. If you were a natural leader then, you are probably in charge in your present role. Shy, diffident, and reluctant to take center stage—is that you now? You can't change your genes or conditioning, but you can make subtle changes to make life more rewarding.

CASE STUDY: CHARLIE

Charlie's mother had conceived him with a lover; her husband guessed, but said nothing for years. His mother disappeared with her lover when Charlie was 6 years old. Then the mental cruelty began. Charlie was excluded without explanation from family meals and ordered to eat in the kitchen. He would listen to his brother and sisters enjoying the same food in the dining room.

All alone in his isolation and bewildered by his father's behavior, he could form no attachment to any older sibling: the other children were forced by their father not to speak to him. At least there was a cook/housekeeper in those days. She provided Charlie with essential affection.

One night, he dreamed of being in a new setting with a wife and two children. They were happy and companionable in a bright, sunlit house. He wrote the dream down and kept it as a talisman for the next 20 years. Charlie's dream came true. The explicit encouragement from its intensely vivid scene gave him the strength to pursue what he most wanted—and deserved.

WOODEN TOYS

Toys made of wood have a special magic for children. They are tactile and solid and usually painted in appealing colors. No wonder some toys have become collector's items since the last century, such is their lasting charm. When they appear in dreams, they can symbolize good times in the past or highlight issues you need to consider in the present.

HAMMERING PEGS INTO ROUND HOLES

Dreaming of sorting discarded toys, you find a wooden hammer-and-pegs game. You remember how children love to bang the round pegs into the holes once they've understood the need to hit hard enough. There's something about that whole-hearted hammering that appeals to you in the dream, and you wake up smiling.

Action About what—or to whom—would you like to hammer home an emotional or political point? You were attracted to the intense movement in the dream: consider what lies behind this and take the hint. Your psyche is encouraging you to make your feelings known in the right quarters—or hole.

YOU FIND ANCESTORS' TOYS

You see an old-fashioned store and go inside: it's a toystore selling antique dolls and playthings. Somehow you know the ones you especially like once belonged to your ancestors. You buy them to take home to give to children, familiar or otherwise. You want to perpetuate the fun you and your ancestors once enjoyed.

Action Understand that finding links with the distant past is important. If possible, trace who your ancestors were, what they did, and what characteristics you inherited from them. Those toys are symbolic of good times you all must have shared. Your psyche is indicating that it's time to start the search.

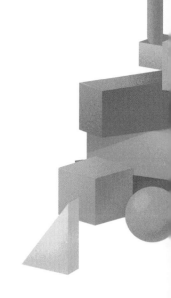

YOU SEE A WOODEN PUPPET UNABLE TO MOVE

In a frightening dream, you see a wooden puppet that seems paralyzed despite its strings. Someone is trying to lift its limbs unsuccessfully from the manipulating platform above. You feel a sense of horror at its inability to respond and shout to try to bring it to life.

Action The puppet on a string is you. Are you in a stuck position in life, unable to move? Who might the puppet master be? Is there a parallel there with someone in your day-to-day routine? Take heart from your act of shouting to try to bring the puppet to life—you are capable of making changes.

COLORED BUILDING BRICKS

Brightly colored wooden bricks tumble out of a toy basket, ready to be built into towers, pretend houses, and walls—hundreds of them, far more than a child could need. There's something deeply attractive about these bricks: you begin to play with them at once, as if you are still a child, building the foundations of a new home.

Action Are you wanting to move or maybe change careers? Building foundations has powerful symbolism: colored bricks would suggest a long-held childhood wish to create something wonderful. Check out the imagery—do primary-colored squares have any present-day significance for you? There is a clue in the dream, and you are invited to decode it.

TRUST IN DREAMS, FOR IN THEM IS HIDDEN THE GATE TO ETERNITY.

KHALIL GIBRAN
THE PROPHET

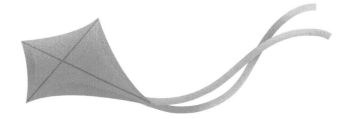

TOYS COMING ALIVE

There are many animated films that suggest fantasy means fun, though some filmmakers choose to morph the inanimate into malevolent living creatures as entertainment. Fun or fearful, the concept of toy characters coming alive is compelling. Their appearance in your dreams is significant and can help identify current emotional problems.

TOYS ARE BEHAVING BADLY

Toys are acting out in your dream in ways that puzzle you. They are behaving in inappropriate ways, such as slashing tires or breaking windows. You watch bewildered as they go about breaking down existing fixtures and making others angry.

Action Reflect on what it is that you want to end or destroy. Is it a tired relationship or a friendship that irritates you? Consider your dream narrative: those toys are at least doing want they want. You might have to make changes by taking drastic measures.

TOYS LIVING YOUR FANTASY LIFE

Your dream takes you to incredible, magical places—to the height of fantastic imagination. Toys come alive and act as you yourself would like to be; adventurous, sociable, entertaining. You identify with their every move and envy their freedom.

Action What are you wanting to make come true in your life? Explore possibilities to help bring more lively company into your world. Those toys represent a subpersonality of yours that is currently being suppressed. Why might this be? What can bring you out of dwelling in a life of fantasy only?

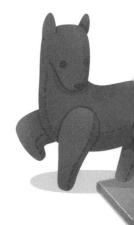

A FRIEND'S TOYS BULLY YOURS

You are back in childhood and enjoying playing with your best friend. To your horror, the friend's toys are bullying yours. You hate what they're doing and want to run home. You feel your toys' imagined suffering.

Action Take a look back to your young days and remember any friends who bossed you around. Did any one person have too much influence over you? Your dream is urging you to let these memories fill you now—and to make up your mind never to let anyone have unhealthy power over you again.

YOUR FAVORITE TOY COMES ALIVE

Your favorite soft toy comes alive, and you greet them in the dream like a long-lost friend. You and the toy once enjoyed wonderful times together, and here you are again, both playing the same games and laughing at the fun.

Action This is wishful thinking, of course: you'd like to curl up and return to childhood. Present worries would disappear if you could permanently recreate this lovely scene. But tempting as it seems, you cannot go back. Acknowledge your wish to return to carefree days, shrug, and get on with the day.

BACK TO SCHOOL

School is all about learning not only the three Rs, but also how to get along with other children. If those school-day experiences weren't the best—through bullying, exclusion, or rejection—this paves the way for difficulties in adulthood. On the other hand, happy times could forecast a more robust future. Learning how to make it so might come through in a dream.

YOU ARE PLAYING GAMES AT SCHOOL

This is a fun dream, full of laughter and joy. Your best friend is there, messing around in the classroom and making you giggle uncontrollably, which is wonderfully freeing.

Action Nostalgia may be just what you're needing right now! Enjoy the memory of that dream, prepare yourself, and get on with the day.

YOU ARE BACK AT SCHOOL WITH ADULTS

You are in a classroom surrounded by adults who are strangers. You are curious about what they are doing, and you want to join in whatever it is that absorbs them. What are they learning? Maybe you notice they are using their hands in some way, enjoying another form of education.

Action A need is being flagged up here to get more stimulation into your life. Consider taking up a new hobby and see that learning a new skill can be richly rewarding.

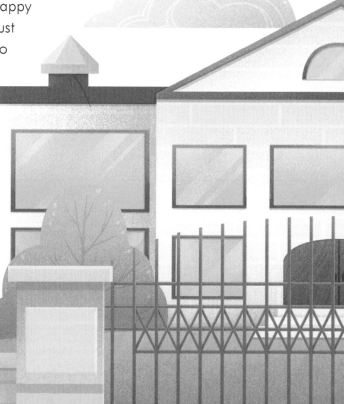

CHILDREN ARE BULLYING SOMEONE

The dream shows a crowd of schoolchildren bullying another child—you realize the child's distress is like your own when you went to school. You feel impotent rage the bullies can't hear your shouts, just like they ignored your crying back then.

Action Those distressing scenes show you why you empathize with victims—on television, in film, or on the street—and do what you can to help. Be glad earlier pain makes you alert to the pain of others and turn your childhood powerlessness into a force for good. Beware of unwelcome interfering: you might get more bullying.

A FELLOW PUPIL IS TERRIFYING YOU

This dream is not so much about children bullying on the playground but of one particular person who terrifies you. They seem like a menacing figure who terrifies the neighborhood, ready with a knife or punch at the slightest provocation—they remind you of a domineering teacher you once knew. You try to run away from school in case you are their next target.

Action Ask yourself who is the menacing person in your present life? They may unwittingly behave in an overpowering way without realizing your fear. Determine to speak to them—you may be pleasantly surprised by their response.

YOU GO TO SCHOOL AS AN ADULT

You are walking through the school doors as an adult yet you're dressed in school clothes as you join your peers. This doesn't faze you; you're one of them.

Action Are you still stuck in your childhood emotionally? Was life in the past much easier than it is now? Accept you are a grown-up with adult responsibilities and be thankful for that dream hint.

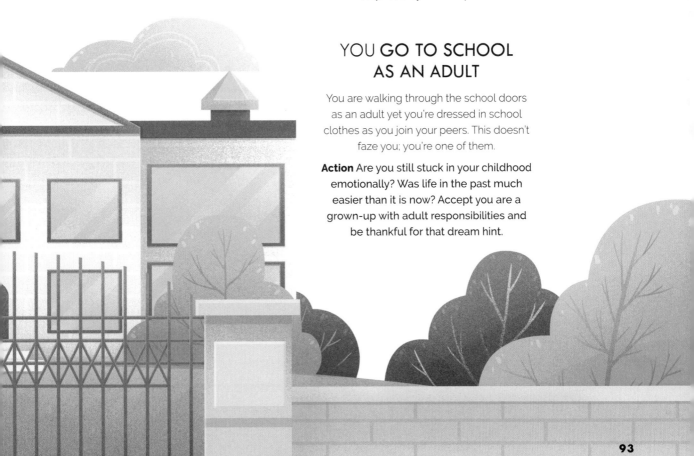

A CLOSET

A closet tells us a good deal about its owner. It holds our clothes, shoes, and hints at our identity. Anyone opening its door could guess quite a lot about the owner. Small wonder closets and wardrobes figure in magical books and in our dreams.

A NARNIA FANTASY DREAM

You find yourself at the back of a huge closet, just like in C. S. Lewis's children's fantasy story. Pushing the clothes to one side, you notice a secret door and open it. A whole new world appears, colorful and inviting. You long to explore but know you cannot.

Action Accept that you might be wanting to escape the real world at the moment. Comfort yourself with the fact that you'd like to climb through a magic door into a better place. Find the courage to face the present difficulties and wait for change that will surely happen.

PRESENTS ARE PILED AT THE TOP OF THE CLOSET

Exciting gift-wrapped presents are glimpsed at the top of the closet. Are they for you, or surely more likely for other people? Wonderful potential is hidden inside the wrapping paper, but you can't believe that richness is destined for you.

Action Gifts represent loving thoughtfulness and the giver wanting you to have the pleasure of accepting them. Are you aware how of much you are loved and appreciated? Reflect on why you doubt their affection. Learn to accept the gift of their feelings, and stop wondering if those closet presents are planned for others.

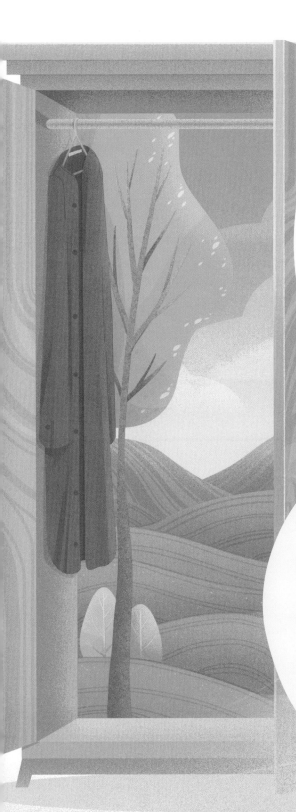

CLOTHES **ARE JAMMED ON THE RACKS**

A dream closet seems ridiculously overfull: clothes are jammed in so tightly it's virtually impossible to pull any one garment out. You struggle to release just one because you need to wear it, but your efforts are useless.

Action Have you taken on a crazy amount of obligations and begun to realize you can't cope? Then make decisions now to offload as many as is reasonable. The pressure you're experiencing is mirrored by the dream—the stress here can mean loss of well-being, or signify future difficulties to face in addition to the load you are already carrying.

THE **CLOSET IS EMPTY**

Standing in an empty room is an empty closet. Forlorn, you pull one door open and feel its emptiness as an emotional blow. Does it remind you of a life that has past? Is the emptiness mirroring your current feelings?

Action That sense of a void in the dream is reflecting a need to consider ways to fill the gap in your life. An empty closet is a metaphor for your sadness, or even depression. Resolve to turn this around, if possible—plan how to change the voids you are experiencing. Perhaps you would find nourishment in following a more spiritual path.

SOMETHING IN THE ATTIC

Attics can mean secrets, outdated keepsakes, or discarded junk. In psychological terms, attics symbolize the mind—that part of the body nearest to the spiritual world. When they appear in our dreams, they have much to say, depending on the context.

TERMITES

You discover your attic's roof timbers have termites and are concerned that, if left untreated, those timbers will suffer serious damage. You imagine the roof collapsing, affecting the whole house, and consider what the astronomical cost will be in undertaking the treatment of those timbers before it is too late.

Action Identify what destructive activity is going on—either in your home or within yourself. The rotting timbers are a metaphor that suggests you need to take steps to protect yourself or your home life in some way. Have you neglected your relationships? Have you failed to notice either someone else's needs or your own? Examine your interaction with others and see how you might be failing to notice a rotten situation, then set about rectifying it before the emotional rot spreads, affecting all concerned.

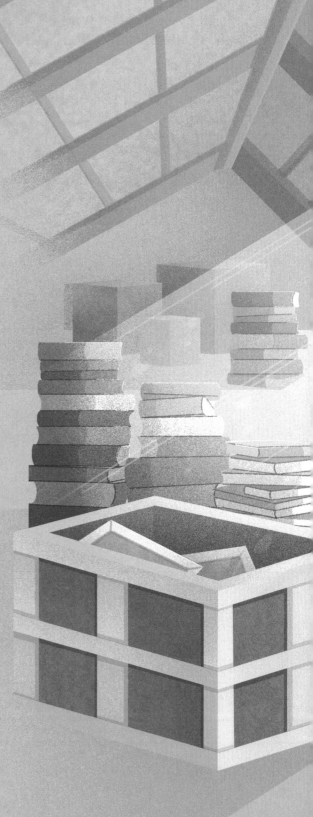

A FAMILY
HISTORY ALBUM

In the dream, you are searching for a mislaid item stored in the attic when you accidentally find an old family album. You discover family secrets you'd never known about and realize one person in particular had a more negative influence on your understanding of these than you had ever appreciated.

Action Ask yourself why this person had such an impact. Isn't it time to alter your perceptions of them? The family myth could have painted a false picture into which—as a young person— you once innocently bought. Now you can evaluate for yourself, make up your own mind about how to see this person, and live your life by your own rules, not following the family's party line.

UNKNOWN
DIARIES

You dream of wandering through a big attic. It has unfamiliar boxes, files, and writings. You search for their provenance, but all you find are unknown people's handwritten diaries. Sitting down on a dusty chest, you read through these autobiographical pages. You see such sadness and so many poignant words that you begin to weep—you want to hold them close forever.

Action If you have never considered writing, take this dream as a hint. Someone else's eloquence—wherever it came from—moved you. Think about using some part of their story or copying the quality of the writing you brought into waking life and try creating a story of your own that honors the original writer.

EMPTY OLD HOUSES

An empty house attracts attention because of its isolation. Does nobody want to live there? Has someone died? Who will be next to bring vitality into the house and nurture it back to life? Dreaming about empty houses is often about the unknown.

YOU WANDER THROUGH EMPTY ROOMS

The front door of an empty house attracts you. Wandering through its rooms, you notice some are furnished, while others are not. Intrigued, you realize this is a big house with several empty rooms. Their forlorn state saddens you, and you want to put furniture, warm drapes, and pictures throughout these bleak quarters.

Action The house is *you*, representing how you are currently feeling. Have you not yet discovered what you're capable of achieving—are there only half-formed ideas around? Your creativity needs expression. Those empty rooms must be furnished psychologically with color and warmth. Accept that you've got everything it takes to transform them.

THE **HOUSE LOOKS** NEGLECTED

An old house looks not only empty but also uncared for. You walk toward it, aware of the peeling paint on the windows. As you put the key in the front door, you turn the latch and step inside. The whole place is in need of attention.

Action Because the house is a metaphor for *you*, understand you need to pay more attention to yourself and take responsibility for it. Consider how much you may have been inattentive—realize you can't burn the candle at both ends. There's a warning here: though you hold the key, you don't yet seem to be opening the door to a better life.

UNDISCOVERED **WINGS**

Inside an empty old house, you're surprised to see a door leading to beautiful rooms unknown to you. You go through and find a new wing leading off the main house. It has many other doors, and you peek inside. The rooms are all empty, and you know that the space is yours.

Action Unknown wings in a house mean your psyche is nudging you to realize your full potential: don't ignore it! Check to see if you are using all of your talents instead of complacently leaving those gifts in the background. Your dream is telling you the time is now, so start manifesting your creativity and furnish those rooms—they aren't yet complete.

UNCOMFORTABLE EMPTINESS

Standing in an empty old house, you know it has been lived in by dozens of people in days gone by. It still retains signs of its previous owners, such as marks on the walls. But now it all feels lifeless, the vitality gone. It seems to mirror your own sense of emptiness.

Action Consider what characteristics contribute to your own emptiness. The house—you—needs to be filled with new life. Resolve to change your attitudes or habits and watch how that void lessens in time when you've taken up an exciting new hobby, study, or friendship.

BURNING HOUSES

There's always a terrible sense of danger when we see or hear about burning houses. Was anyone hurt in the fire? Was the house completely gutted? They can also mean danger for those who try to put out the flames. Dreams tend to reflect these elements of risk and courage.

YOU ARE WATCHING A HOUSE BURNING

You are witnessing a terrible house fire and stand by listlessly as it burns down. The firefighters arrive and set to work while you stand aside, unconcerned for anyone carried outside who might need your support.

Action What are you doing in your life that's causing such distancing? Does that lack of concern for others also apply to your inability to take care of yourself? Because the house is on fire—and it represents you—examine what might be the cause of your life going up in flames. Be the firefighter and find the courage to stop it from doing anymore damage.

YOU ARE THROWING THE PAST INTO THE FLAMES

As a fire is raging in a house across the street, you run into your own property and look for notebooks hidden in a desk. Your own house is safe, but there are compromising notes you want to take outside and commit to the flames across the road. You find your notebooks and hurl them thankfully into the fire.

Action What do you need to let go? Did you write about anger in the pages—anger you suppressed or kept hidden? It's time to release pent-up rage rather than allow it to continue to disturb you. Committing powerful words to the flames is a useful ritual in real life.

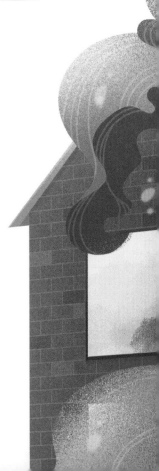

YOU ADMIRE THE FIREFIGHTERS' BRAVERY

You are watching the fire engines arrive and firefighters efficiently set about controlling the flames. The burning house is a tall one, with many windows through which flames are already emerging. Firefighters climb up ladders—they face serious danger, and you admire their courage.

Action How timid are you? Would that kind of physical bravery be beyond you, or are you ready to be more courageous in your social life? The scenario is showing you others' ability to face difficult situations: it's a timely message to consider how to emulate that approach.

THE HOUSE IS COMPLETELY DESTROYED

A burning house collapses to the ground, completely destroyed by the fire. You watch in horror: no one has been hurt, but the sight is shocking. What once held boisterous families, pets, and noise is now a heap of ashes. You wonder what will become of the land.

Action This is a dream about death and renewal. Accept the need in your life for the new—for radical change. The collapse of the house represents collapse of your own sense of self, but this is a positive move. Your psyche is hinting at new growth that will eventually arise from those ashes.

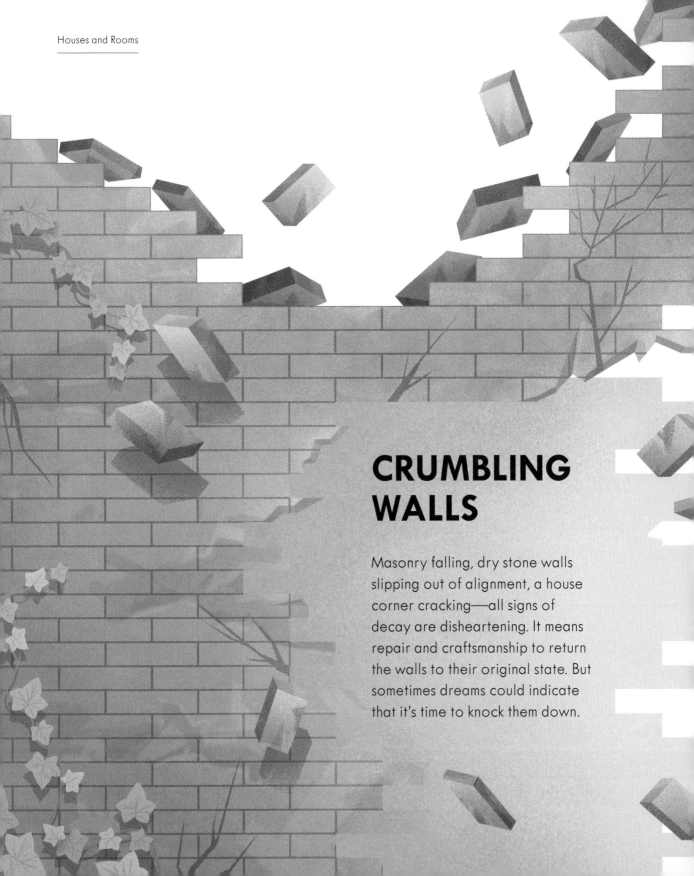

CRUMBLING WALLS

Masonry falling, dry stone walls slipping out of alignment, a house corner cracking—all signs of decay are disheartening. It means repair and craftsmanship to return the walls to their original state. But sometimes dreams could indicate that it's time to knock them down.

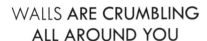

WALLS ARE CRUMBLING ALL AROUND YOU

This is a bleak dream where you see walls all around you crumbling and even falling. Every time you try to shore up a wall, you hear another begin to collapse. You run upstairs to see what might be happening on the first floor, aghast to see big cracks on the corner of exterior walls. You dread seeing that the roof has been affected, too. But those timbers are in good condition, as are the roof tiles as far as you can tell. You wake up, exhausted at the potential work involved.

Action If you have been feeling depressed lately, accept that, though bleak, this dream is reflecting your state of mind at the moment. Note that the top of the house, symbolizing your mental state, is in good condition. Take comfort from that information, but consider the good sense in booking an appointment with your doctor or alternative health practitioner to help you restore the balance needed to support your metaphorical house. You need a boost to help you feel more buoyant.

YOUR GARDEN WALL IS CRUMBLING

While working in your garden, you suddenly notice an old wall is crumbling to the point of being useless. Scavengers can come and go, so your garden harvest is at risk of being spoiled or eaten.

Action The dream garden wall is your personal boundary—and it's not being carefully guarded. You need to pay attention to containing all of your hard efforts. Resolve to examine your boundary attitudes. You may be letting human pests of one kind or another into your personal space too freely.

CONCERN ABOUT THE FOUNDATIONS

There's a serious crack appearing in a corner of your house. In the dream, you realize this can only mean one thing—the foundations have shifted. Desperately, you run around the exterior and see another corner of the house shows the telltale signs, too.

Action This might be a metaphor for a crumbling foundation to a relationship or work situation. Do not despair: this comes as a warning to pay attention (as you did in the dream) to the danger signs. Restoration is necessary! Set to and work out what needs your careful consideration to avert the current potential crisis.

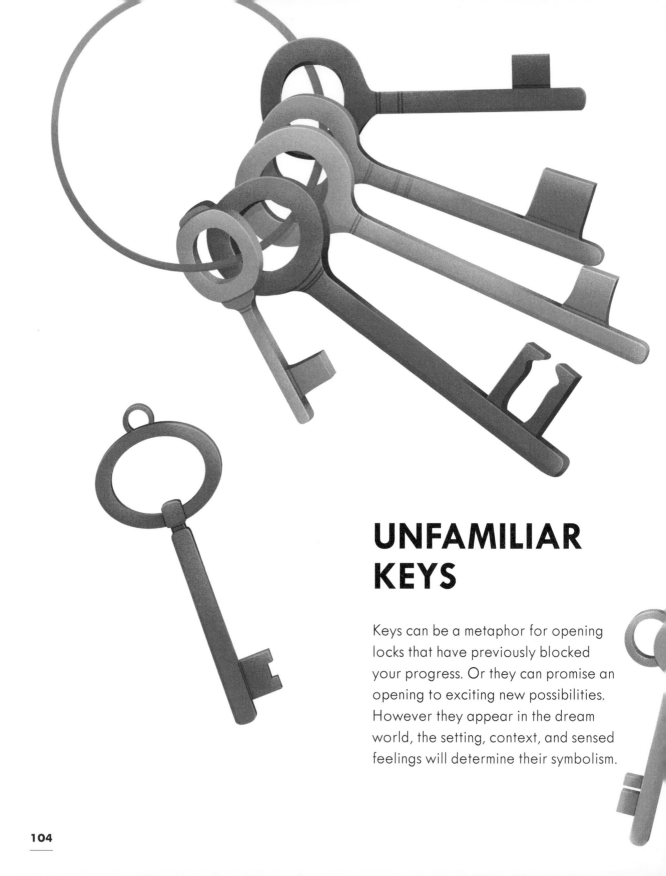

UNFAMILIAR KEYS

Keys can be a metaphor for opening locks that have previously blocked your progress. Or they can promise an opening to exciting new possibilities. However they appear in the dream world, the setting, context, and sensed feelings will determine their symbolism.

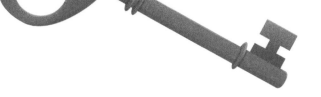

THE **KEYS MAKE YOU FEEL UNCOMFORTABLE**

You see a bunch of strange, unfamiliar keys. You have no idea where they might fit in your present home or workplace. They seem to be significant, and you wish you could place exactly why. Obviously old enough to belong to the distant past, those keys make you feel uncomfortable.

Action Consider what they might represent. What is it you should unlock in your memory, hidden from your conscious mind? Perhaps it is time now to turn the key and remember the reason for your discomfort. Maybe looking through old photographs or letters might help bring the memories to the surface. Tell yourself you are grown up now; you can cope.

THE **KEY DOESN'T FIT IN THE LOCK**

A key that you somehow know once closed the door on a chance to change your life for the better has appeared in a dream. You grieve as you look at this key and wish you could somehow use it again to open that door. But putting it into the lock eludes you. It just won't fit.

Action Realize the dream key is no longer the right one. If it did once hold the answer to a lost opportunity, accept its loss. But a key is still within you—you are capable of making other opportunities come your way. What are your gifts? Decide to use them to reach your full potential.

AN **ANCIENT IRON KEY TO AN OLD DOOR**

A massive ancient key, ornate and heavy, has been placed on a table. You want to see what it might unlock—then an old oak door appears from nowhere. You put the key in its lock and feel cautious when it turns. The door opens to a vaulted hall, home of forgotten esoteric mysteries. You feel diffident, yet somehow you know you're invited to explore.

Action Remember how wary you felt in this dream. Does that reflect your reluctance to venture into new territory in real life? Rewarding discoveries may await you, but only if you calm your fears.

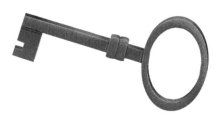

SKELETONS **BEHIND THE LOCKED DOOR**

You open a forbidden door with an unfamiliar key and see piles of skeletons. You slam the door shut and run away as fast as you can. The scary scene of all those bones haunts you when you wake up.

Action What are the skeletons behind your door? Trust your psyche; it is showing that you must take a further look at those stored memories. If you feel you need help, discuss the secrets with qualified people. Once released in those discussions, those skeletons could take on an entirely new perspective.

SEARCHING FOR THE BATHROOM

We must all use the bathroom for the natural elimination of body waste. Waste matter is a metaphor for our psychological urine and feces: the stored material influencing our responses to life. Dreams of this kind often illustrate the need for release.

YOU ARE ANGRY IN YOUR SEARCH

In your dream, you are feeling very angry and you need a bathroom, but you cannot find one. There is no safe place to expel your feces, so you hold the bowel movement in while your anger builds up to bursting point. You feel desperate in your predicament, and your anger seems to blur with the fury at the lack of a suitable place.

Action Ask yourself: why do you need to hold back your anger? Find out what it's all about, then decide either to release it—if it would be helpful—or keep quiet.

YOU FEAR EMBARRASSMENT

A dream takes you from room to room, never finding the right door to a bathroom. Your need is increasingly urgent, and you become alarmed at the prospect of an embarrassing accident on the floor. You dread the shame of anyone witnessing the scene.

Action Be aware of your dread of shaming yourself in public or even in front of just one person. Cast your mind back to childhood—were your parents likely to have shown disgust at a dirty diaper or others' dirt? This often lies behind a present dread. It will take determination, but try to accept the fact that accidents happen.

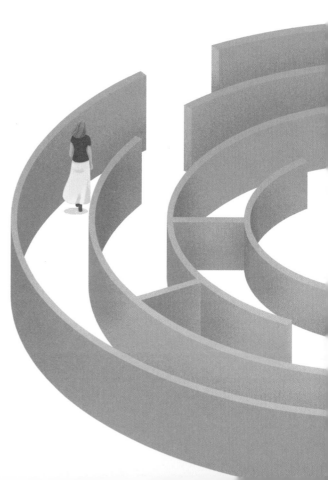

THE DREAM SEARCH IS PRIMAL

The search for a bathroom is desperate: you can't find one. You know it's important, but bewilderingly it doesn't seem to be to relieve your bladder. You then see a cat urinate against a bush, marking its territory, and feel an instinctual connection to what the cat is doing.

Action What territory do you need to mark in your life? Is another person interested in your partner, taking your job, or stealing your friends? Consider how best you can protect your interests.

CASE STUDY: AMY

Amy was a young teenager whose parents innocently left her for a week in the care of a close male friend, a lonely widower. The widower was a predator. He promised Amy gifts and kissed her inappropriately, declaring his love for her. She was frightened of him and his insistence that she keep their secret. She decided to tell her parents. Sadly, both failed to see any danger. Amy felt betrayed by all three adults. The widower then turned his attention to Amy's mother, with Dad often away on business. Fights and denials followed, as her father became increasingly worried his wife would leave him. He suffered the first of three heart attacks, the last one killing him.

Amy carried her fury into middle age. One night, she dreamed of searching for the bathroom but not finding one. A child's potty appeared, and she urinated into that before carrying it to the top of the stairs. The widower (long deceased) was walking below in the hall. She poured her urine satisfyingly on top of his head. At last, all her pent-up emotions had found release. When Amy woke, she laughed with glee—and then wept some necessary healing tears.

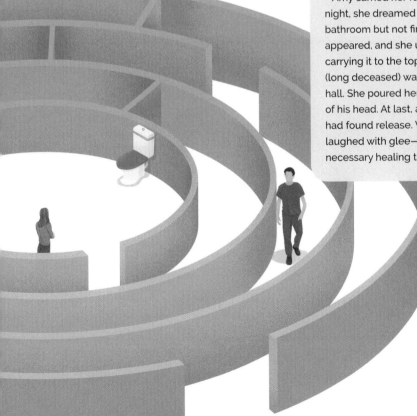

DRIVING

Driving is the means by which we go from one place to another. A vehicle of some sort conveys driver and passengers comfortably from house to house, providing transportation with the least inconvenience. But driving can mean trouble—if the person at the controls is not paying attention—and dreams often point this out.

YOU **ARE DRIVING DANGEROUSLY**

You dream of driving your car haphazardly, taking too many risks. Speeding along, you get a buzz from the thrill of it and have no thought about any possible danger to yourself or others.

Action If the dream activity is the opposite of your day-to-day driving habits, then consider this a wish fulfillment—it's certainly safer to drive fast in your sleep. If it mirrors what you enjoy doing in real life, then stop! Cool down and be more responsible.

YOU ARE CAUGHT IN A TRAFFIC JAM

The dream has you waiting impatiently in a traffic jam. The minutes tick by, with no sign of movement ahead. Frustrated, you won't keep an appointment and have no means of letting anyone know you will be late.

Action Accept that blockages happen. You need to learn to wait patiently for those life blocks to disappear—as they surely will in the end. Consider that you are being made to stop, as in the dream, for a reason. Cast your mind back to those times when you strongly thought one thing, only to change your view after events had unfolded. Learn from that observation.

YOU ARE FACING THE OPEN ROAD

Car keys in hand, your meeting satisfactorily completed, you start the engine and set off down the highway. You rejoice in your freedom, facing the open road with that successful appointment outcome no longer your responsibility. The road is traffic-free and you roll along, feeling great.

Action Congratulate yourself on having done a competent job—whatever it is you've been doing recently. You deserve a rest, so perhaps plan a break.

YOU ARE STEERING FROM THE BACK SEAT

Controlling the car from the back seat—literally holding the steering wheel from behind the driver's seat—you are uncomfortable and afraid. You long to stop the car, but of course your leg can't reach the brake pedal.

Action Check out the impossible positions you tend to put yourself in at home or at work—and about the relationships you form outside those. What makes you put yourself into such dangerous situations? Resolve to end this risky habit. It will eventually cause an accident of some kind.

A PUNCTURE HALTS YOUR JOURNEY

In your dream, your steering wheel wobbles; it's a tire puncture, and you're in the fast lane. Drivers honk as you aim dangerously for the side of the road. You're frightened and discover you've forgotten your smartphone. Someone then pulls up behind your car to help you, and thankfully you set off again.

Action You're not alone. You don't have to deal with every crisis on your own. Trust that help *does* turn up when it's most needed.

FLYING

Dreams about flying are usually enjoyable—soaring through the sky or skimming over the earth's surface can mean a longing for freedom and self-empowerment. Alternatively, you may feel terrified. Reflecting on the emotions felt in your dream will help you better understand its message.

YOU **WANT TO FLY AWAY**

You want to escape and fly away by your own magical efforts to the great blue yonder. You have a wonderful time, flying higher and higher. You then dive down and see your home far below you. Suddenly the flying has lost its fun factor.

Action Ask yourself why you want to leave home and escape from a more grounded life. Can you not stay the course and wait for change? Fleeing from responsibilities or emotional problems may not be the answer that best serves your development.

YOU'RE **FLYING TOO CLOSE TO THE SUN**

The dream is taking you so high, you begin to feel the sun's warmth a little too fiercely. You are flying all by yourself, strongly and completely confident in your own powers to fly without an engine. You are possibly in danger, but you believe you are immortal.

Action Remember Icarus, whose father Daedalus warned him not to fly too close to the sun for fear that his wax wings would melt. Full of hubris, Icarus ignored the warning and perished. Can you acknowledge some inflation in a subpersonality you may have? Work on it or suffer the consequences.

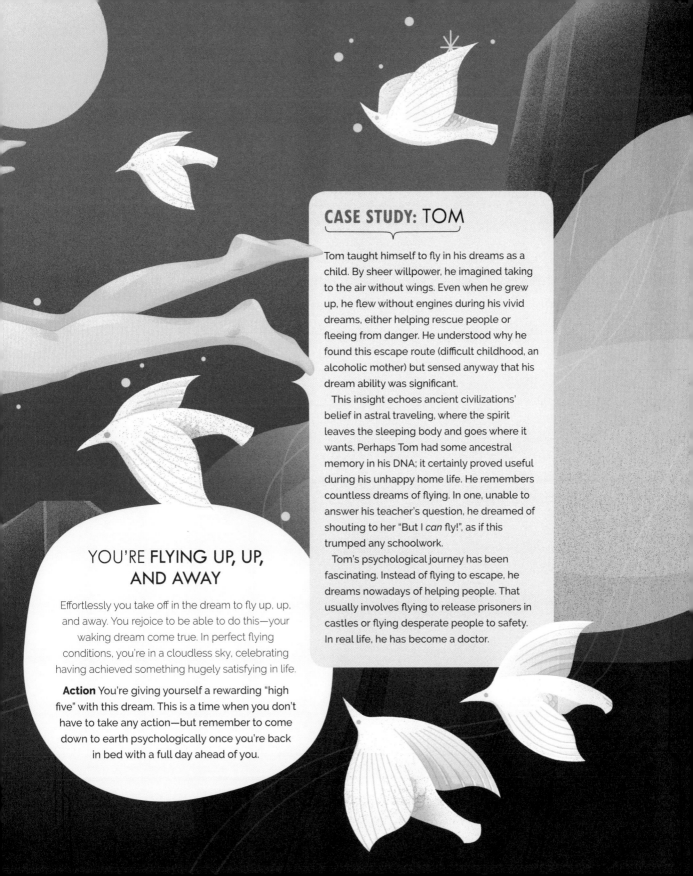

CASE STUDY: TOM

Tom taught himself to fly in his dreams as a child. By sheer willpower, he imagined taking to the air without wings. Even when he grew up, he flew without engines during his vivid dreams, either helping rescue people or fleeing from danger. He understood why he found this escape route (difficult childhood, an alcoholic mother) but sensed anyway that his dream ability was significant.

This insight echoes ancient civilizations' belief in astral traveling, where the spirit leaves the sleeping body and goes where it wants. Perhaps Tom had some ancestral memory in his DNA; it certainly proved useful during his unhappy home life. He remembers countless dreams of flying. In one, unable to answer his teacher's question, he dreamed of shouting to her "But I *can* fly!", as if this trumped any schoolwork.

Tom's psychological journey has been fascinating. Instead of flying to escape, he dreams nowadays of helping people. That usually involves flying to release prisoners in castles or flying desperate people to safety. In real life, he has become a doctor.

YOU'RE FLYING UP, UP, AND AWAY

Effortlessly you take off in the dream to fly up, up, and away. You rejoice to be able to do this—your waking dream come true. In perfect flying conditions, you're in a cloudless sky, celebrating having achieved something hugely satisfying in life.

Action You're giving yourself a rewarding "high five" with this dream. This is a time when you don't have to take any action—but remember to come down to earth psychologically once you're back in bed with a full day ahead of you.

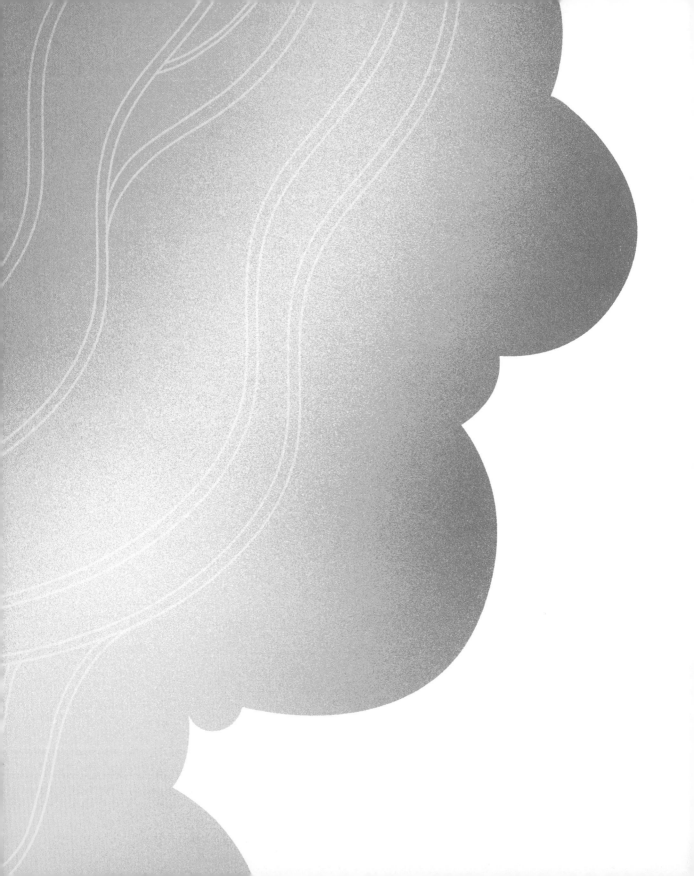

> DON'T BE PUSHED BY
> YOUR PROBLEMS; BE LED
> BY YOUR DREAMS.

RALPH WALDO EMERSON
THE JOURNALS AND NOTEBOOKS

TRANSPORTATION

Riverboats, walking or riding, flying, or going by train are all interesting topics for the dreamer—even if we have no conscious choice in the subject. Going from A to B has a certain energy about it: it is a journey, whether actual or emotional. Dreams about traveling often indicate a psychological movement toward change of some sort.

A TURBULENT BOAT RIDE

You dream of being aboard a boat in rough waters. Huge waves threaten to engulf you, and the boat's rolling is making you feel seasick. The water is frighteningly deep, yet you feel in no particular danger. Instead, you feel a sense of resignation at having to go through this ordeal.

Action Waves are bringing up to your conscious mind an issue you've been ignoring. Ask yourself: what emotional issue have you been pushing away? The deeper the water, the deeper the unexpressed acknowledgment of your wish not to be overwhelmed by it. So what recent event has triggered this dream? Start putting two and two together.

YOU ARE ESCAPING ON A HANDMADE RAFT

You find yourself on a desert island and are appalled at your isolation. You want to get home, so you set to work finding logs and twine to make a raft. Once afloat out on the open ocean, your next worry is about the logs—they seem to be separating, and the twine is untying itself. You fear you might have made a catastrophic mistake leaving.

Action Your anxiety is about achieving a transition safely, but have you thought you might not actually want to leave, be it home, your job, or a relationship? Quiz yourself on whether you are ready to consider a departure. Is this the right time?

THE PILOT IS BEING MALICIOUS

The plane ride on which you are a passenger gets very bumpy. You begin to wonder if the pilot is playing games with the passengers, abusing his or her all-powerful control by taking reckless and unnecessary risks.

Action The pilot is you, the dreamer: what risks are *you* taking? Identify the abusive part of yourself that is happy to alarm people. Do you dislike an aspect of yourself, that casual thoughtlessness—are you aware that this is how you behave sometimes? If so, it is certainly time to consider your behavior and how it affects the people you love.

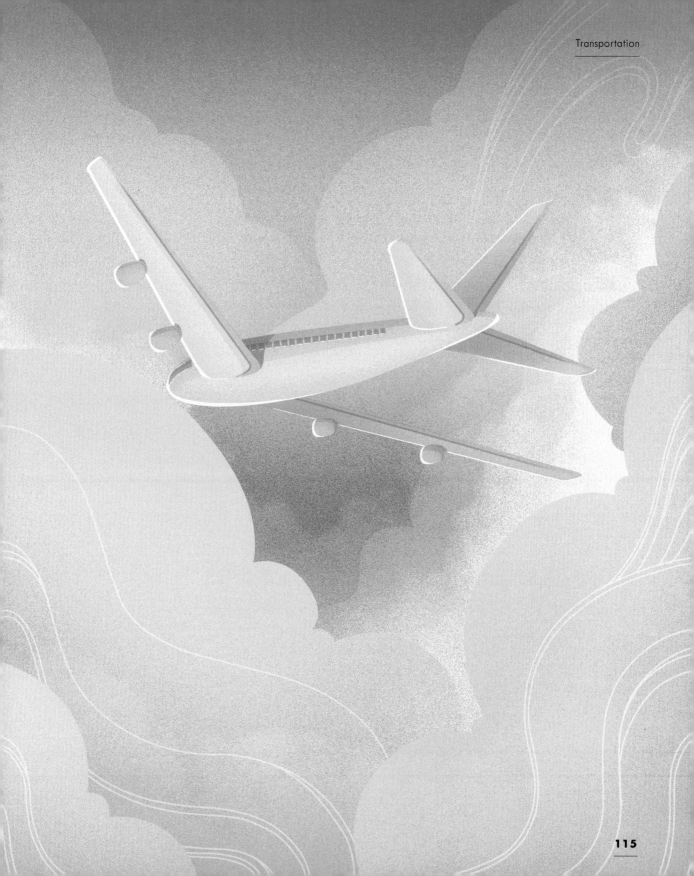

ACCIDENTS

Accidents usually mean distress, anxiety, and pain. Dreams about them often mirror our current feelings: a sense of impending doom and a tensing against a crash of some kind, whether the hard impact is literal or emotional. Dreams of accidents play out our fears—or sometimes warn of the avoidable.

A **HIGHWAY TRAFFIC ACCIDENT**

You are driving along and see a bad accident on the other side of the highway. Ambulances and police cars surround the scene, and you are full of concern about the outcome for the drivers and passengers involved. There is nothing you can do; you must speed on in the opposite direction.

Action This is an anxiety dream about strangers colliding in all senses with those you love, causing distress to everyone. As in the dream, there is nothing appropriate for you to do—you must let others make their mistakes. Therein lie the lessons they must learn.

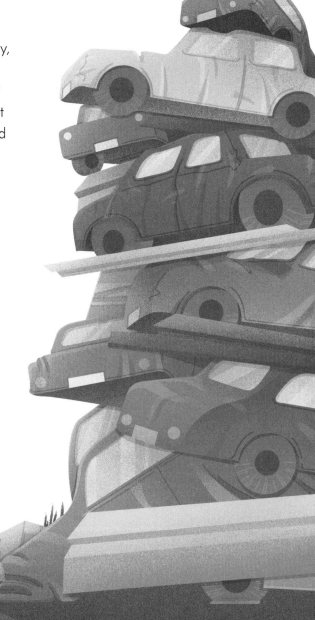

YOUR FLIGHT IS DELAYED

The runway has closed following an accident, and you miss your flight. In your dream, the delay goes on interminably, but you don't lose your cool and sit down with a coffee and a book to wait for developments. While other passengers are shouting angrily, you get absorbed in your book, resigned at missing an urgent appointment.

Action Celebrate your calm acceptance of the way life is turning out. Delays happen, and you have learned to see difficult situations through, knowing movement will happen when all the pieces are in place.

A BIKE PILE-UP

You are cycling with friends, negotiating hairpin turns and speeding recklessly downhill. You feel powerful, like a winner, despite there being no competition. But suddenly you take the next turn too sharply, causing a terrible pile-up. Your friends fall off, screaming in pain as they hit the pavement. You alone are responsible—leading them, you took a foolish chance.

Action A bicycle—a speedy extension of yourself—is a useful metaphor in the dream to warn about taking risks where others will suffer, too. What are you doing too fast and too carelessly? Don't let hubris cause an emotional accident. Approach unseen corners in life with more caution.

YOU RUN INTO A LAMPPOST

You are cycling in town and, losing attention as you look in a store window, run into a lamppost. Passersby either stop to ask if you are hurt or smirk at their friends. You feel annoyed on all counts, particularly as you will be late for work. You wonder what local government you can blame for the lamppost's faulty position.

Action What is it in front of your nose that you are failing to see because your attention wanders? Count the number of times you experience collisions in relationships: is this emotional avoidance or just plain carelessness? Resolve to pay better attention to your everyday behavior, looking for possible distress before it happens. You will be happier this way.

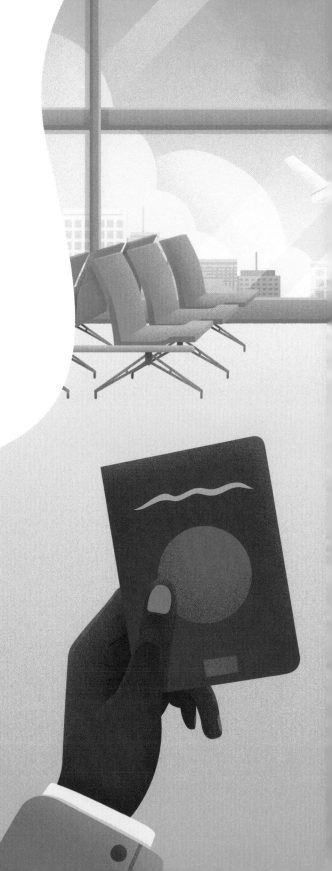

A PASSPORT

A passport is the vital document allowing you to cross frontiers—to travel into another country. It is your identity and the means by which you can go from place to place. Dreams often acknowledge the importance of a passport, but it tends to be a metaphor for something else.

YOUR **PASSPORT IS OUT OF DATE**

A customs officer is scrutinizing your passport and frowning. He hands it back to you, remarking that it's out of date. Your route is blocked. There's no way you can cajole, charm, or bluster your way through.

Action Accept this dream as a sign you can't yet move, whether this means your home, job, or career. Now is not the right time. Do some careful thinking after the dream's obvious hint. Ask yourself what work must first be done on yourself to find out how you can later symbolically make your "passport" current.

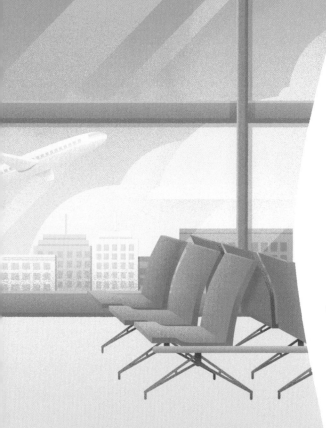

YOU ARE WATCHING OTHER TRAVELERS

You are standing in an airport departure lounge, merely interested as you see hundreds of people waiting for their flight announcement or ready to show their passports at the check-in counter. You are curious about their destinations and wonder what different countries they are flying to, and what lies ahead for them. You then realize you have your own passport in your hand.

Action Key to the message in this dream is your interest and curiosity as you watch others depart for unknown lands. You have the means now to move—your passport is evidence of this—so be encouraged by the positive note to this dream. Additionally, you are psychologically ready to move.

YOUR PASSPORT PHOTO IS OF SOMEONE ELSE

You are among a crowd of travelers lining up at airport arrival counters. They are all holding out their passports for inspection, and you present yours. Then you suddenly realize the photograph in your passport does not show your own face—it's of someone else. You're turned away; you cannot travel.

Action This dream is about how you present yourself to the world. It is clearly time to be more authentic and showed your true self. Understand that even though you may have spent years creating a public image—how you look, dress, speak, and act—your psyche is nudging you to get real. Inauthenticity doesn't work: practice, little by little, letting others see who you really are.

A DECEASED RELATIVE'S PASSPORT

Searching for papers in the drawer of a deceased relative's desk, you chance upon their passport. It's long outdated, and their photograph shows a much younger version of the person you remember. You are surprisingly touched to see that youthful face in the passport.

Action Ask yourself: Why have this dream now? What is going on in life that triggered memories of this relative—were they happy or not so happy? Their hopeful young face might be relevant, or perhaps you need only to reflect on the preciousness of life. Is its message to enjoy what you have?

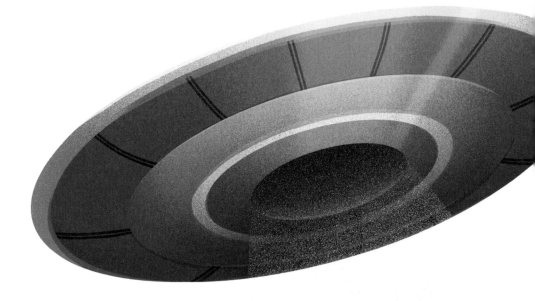

ALIEN SPACECRAFT

Films and television shows have fantasized for decades about visitors from outer space. Websites report countless numbers of people claiming to have been abducted in a spacecraft. The alien phenomenon has landed, and—inevitably—our dreams can reflect this. They are likely to be a metaphor for escape, hint at adventure seeking, or signify curiosity about the universe.

YOU **ARE ABDUCTED BY ALIENS**

Against your will, you are abducted by aliens and taken away in their spaceship. The aliens terrify you with their cold, uncaring behavior. You feel completely powerless, out of control and at their mercy.

Action Look at your down-to-earth situation: Who or what is making you feel so powerless and out of control? Does the aliens' coldness reflect another's uncaring behavior? If the reason lies with someone obvious, talk to a trusted person about what's happening. You might need help to avoid the toxicity.

YOU ARE WALKING ON THE MOON ALL ALONE

You are walking on the surface of the moon, enjoying the freedom of being alone. A spacecraft brought you here and left you on the moon at your request. To your surprise, another spaceship appears with the invitation to hitch a ride back home. You wave the aliens away and watch their craft zoom off. You're pleased to be left alone once again, more than ready to enjoy this new territory.

Action You have probably made a big move in your life—perhaps relocating to another part of the country—and are deciding in this dream to stay put and explore your new environment. Give yourself a pat on the back for that courage to make this life change and settle down to find out more of what the surroundings have to offer.

ALIENS IN THE NEIGHBORHOOD

A spacecraft has suddenly appeared on a piece of land near your home. Its occupants beckon you and your family to join them, and you can't decide in the dream whether to do so. The spaceship is intriguing: you are tempted to explore but hold back.

Action Who are the "aliens" in your life? Is there a different community living nearby about whom you feel suspicious or uneasy? Ask yourself if being friendly with those strangers would be a progressive move—or are you afraid of exploring possibilities? Weigh up the potential here and take appropriate action. You can always withdraw later.

FLEEING TO ANOTHER PLANET

You are traveling in a spaceship going to another planet. Very excited and relieved to be leaving Earth, with all its humdrum activity, you sit back to enjoy the ride. Suddenly, on a screen, you see a close relative weeping because you've left home. You regret your drastic decision.

Action Even if you want to run away from home, consider the impact on those you leave behind. You are conflicted with that need and the awareness of pain you would cause, so talk about it. Admit your unhappiness and try to find a resolution without causing irrevocable damage.

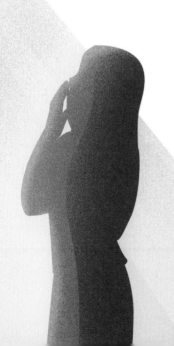

DARK UNDERGROUND PLACES

Dark underground places are metaphors for the unconscious mind. They are the areas most of us least want to explore: fearsome for their unknown terrain, far from the comforting light of day. However, only by exploring those hidden areas—by delving into the unconscious world—can we reach that vital goal of understanding.

ESCAPING THROUGH A DARK UNDERGROUND PASSAGE

You are hurrying down an escape tunnel that is dark and damp. Desperate to get out of this constricting place, you've become increasingly claustrophobic. But you dread being discovered and taken back to wherever it was you escaped from, knowing how punishing that return will inevitably be for you.

Action Is this dream describing how you feel about escaping from a combative situation or partner? Plan your escape and take into account that, though possibly dangerous, there will be the proverbial light at the end of that tunnel once you are sure it is right to try to get away.

EXPLORING A SUBTERRANEAN CAVE

A companion and you are exploring a subterranean cave. At first, it seems like an interesting adventure, and you are both enjoying the eerie sensation of being in this underground passage—it's another world. But you become increasingly uneasy despite the sense of adventure. It's a familiar feeling, and you begin to wish you hadn't started this journey. Yet there's a certainty, too, that there's no going back.

Action Identify that part of you currently feeling ambivalent about your situation. Dark underground places symbolize the world of the unconscious: have you stumbled into exploring your own inner world and feel uneasy about what you may find? Continue your exploration—whether in therapy or with other work—and you will come to grips with that fear.

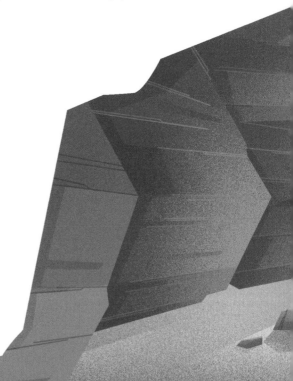

YOU'RE IN AN UNDERGROUND MINE

You find yourself in an old underground passage of a mine. Wandering through its labyrinth of tunnels, you begin to worry about the pollution down there and what danger to others' breathing all this dust and stagnant air must cause. You hurry to get out.

Action Does stagnant air have significance, such as literally representing your working conditions, or perhaps something more subtle back at home? People's repressed emotions can produce the equivalent of stale, almost toxic, air. If this applies to your domestic life, consider measures to emotionally freshen up your environment.

CASE STUDY: JACK

Jack dreamed he was wading in sewer water along with other people in an underground passage. They reached a halfway point where the sewer water stopped and they could rest. He saw lockers on a wall and knew he must leave his keys, wallet, and phone there. As he opened a rusty old locker, he noticed others had left their possessions, too. Was this a rite of passage for travelers? He saw a decaying pile of belongings; their owners clearly hadn't returned to reclaim them. Undaunted by the sinister implication, Jack knew he must carry on with his journey. He walked down the steep passage ahead, deeper and increasingly darker. He knew with absolute certainty now that this passage would eventually turn upward and he'd get out into a happier life.

Later, he understood the dream's message. Jack had long struggled with his relationships, so he went into therapy for help. His dream offered him the confidence to look courageously into his unconscious—underground—world and correctly forecast the outcome.

"

DREAMS ARE
THE TOUCHSTONE OF
OUR CHARACTERS.

"

HENRY D. THOREAU
A WEEK ON THE CONCORD AND MERRIMACK RIVERS

A BRIDGE LEADING TO NOWHERE

There's something scary about a bridge leading to nowhere, accustomed as we are to crossing over a bridge to reach a recognized other side. However, sometimes our psyche requires us to face the unknown, where the destination is a blank. A dream can lead us usefully to do battle with uncertainty.

YOU ARE FINDING THE COURAGE TO CROSS

There is darkness all around, and you are plucking up the courage to step onto an unknown bridge. Your journey has brought you to this threshold, and there's no turning back. You have no idea where this bridge might take you, but somehow you know you must cross it.

Action Courage has been illustrated here—be pleased at your sense of adventure and realize that bridges *must* lead somewhere. Does this apply to an emotional or employment bridge you're contemplating? Take your next steps bravely and remember that the other side is attached as firmly as this side.

BROKEN STEPS TO A BRIDGE

You feel compelled to climb steps up to a bridge, with no idea where that bridge leads. Nearing the top step, you see to your horror that you must first jump over a large hole. For some reason, you cannot turn back—you have to make the jump.

Action Life isn't easy for you at the moment. No sooner do you take the necessary steps for advancement than your next move seems imperiled. See the hole in the steps as the final challenge before you make the brave leap to comparative safety. It may appear to lead nowhere, but this bridge is likely to take you to meet your destiny—you need to find the courage to jump.

NOWHERE BECOMES SOMEWHERE

You cross over a bridge leading to nowhere, hesitating as it sways slightly in the wind and feeling doubtful about carrying on. But you persist with an increasing sense of curiosity. At last, you step onto new territory and walk into unfamiliar surroundings. You like what you see; there's a newness to it all that appeals.

Action Rejoice that you pressed on despite your doubts. Make a mental note of when you decided to set out for new territory: you may need to return across this metaphorical bridge to finish up matters before you go on to experience fully this unexplored chapter.

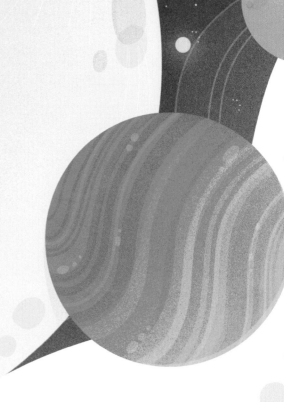

OTHER WORLDS

We are accustomed these days to talking about other galaxies and planets. We also read about or see documentaries on the fascinating concept of space travel and time jumps. The psyche has rich seams to plunder to furnish our dream world: great mysteries yet to be understood but enthralling in their elusiveness.

EXPLORING **ANOTHER WORLD**

Scientifically absorbed, you find yourself on a distant planet doing research. You take scrapings and gaze into a microscope, thrilled at your discoveries. You call out to your colleagues to take a look—but there's no one there. Alone, you're disappointed not to be sharing these marvels.

Action Ask yourself if you are guilty of getting too focused on ideas, leaving everyone behind as you race ahead. Be more aware of when it is appropriate to include others. Explain your behavior: no one likes to be excluded.

EXOTIC **COUNTRIES** BECKON

A street market abroad is the setting for your dream; the aroma of unknown food is enticing as you wander down a street in this sunny new world. You observe people greeting one another with loud, excited exclamations as they make their purchases—quite different from your hometown experience. You want to join them but wonder if you would fit into such a different environment.

Action Are you tempted in reality by the idea of living in faraway lands—the more exotic, the better? From the doubtful note in your dream, perhaps you're not yet ready to embark on such a major change. Consider how best to prepare long term for such a bold move. Your psyche has deliberately given you a preview: be encouraged.

A **FUTURE WORLD**

In your dream, you find yourself in a bleak futuristic landscape. Robots are everywhere, and you see only driverless vehicles. People look like zombies, and the skies are full of strange-looking craft. There is no sign of nature anywhere.

Action There *is* no action to take: you have time traveled in your dream, perhaps as a consequence of worrying about climate change. Enjoy what you can of the world now—that gloomy future may not happen. Your anxiety created this unhappy scene.

CASE STUDY: ALEX

Alex dreamed vividly of walking along a road familiar to him in the countryside and seeing old friends harvesting in the fields. He looked across the rural landscape and there were carthorses, wagons, and men and women in 18th-century clothes, scything and collecting the corn into stacks, ready to load on the wagons. He waved, and two men waved back. That same dream recurred twice more, then stopped. "It was bizarre but felt absolutely real," he said. "I was there in the summer sunshine, could smell the dust from the cut corn and hear the birds."

Weeks before his first dream, Alex had spent several days in the hospital with a concussion after a fall. Had his brain been affected enough to tune him temporarily into another time zone? Interestingly, this is not an unknown phenomenon. There are countless reports of people who vividly dream of being in another century.

129

CROSSROADS

Crossroads in mythology and folklore are magical locations between the worlds, where supernatural spirits can be contacted. More prosaically, they are the point at which roads meet and, psychologically, where important decisions must be made. They often appear in dreams to indicate turning points for the dreamer.

A CRASH AT THE CROSSROADS

A car suddenly crashes into the back of yours while you pause at a crossroads. Surprised, you are being shouted at by the driver of the other car. They claim the accident certainly wasn't their fault—it was yours! They furiously inform you they watched you sitting there for ages when you could have driven on. They had urgent business, now ruined by your inattention.

Action Be more aware of how indecisive you can be. Are you inconveniencing people by your lack of thought for their welfare? Let this dream urge you to examine your attitudes and realize there are behavioral boundaries as well as physical ones, just as at your dream crossroads.

MOONLIGHT OVER CROSSROADS

Standing in the middle of the intersection of two roads, you are of two minds about an emotional problem. It is nighttime, and a full moon casts confusing shadows. You look more closely at the contrast, though you are still not yet sure what to do. The moon's illumination then somehow points out the light and the dark in your moral dilemma. Suddenly, you understand with total clarity which route to take.

Action The moon represents your intuitive feminine aspect, and this dream is guiding you to make the right choice. Be grateful that your psyche seems to have already resolved your problem. It should now be obvious what you must do. However tempting, don't ignore that advice.

CROSSROADS OF INDECISION

You are standing at a busy intersection, bewildered at the choice you must make: which road next? You can't make up your mind and are terrified you will meet with an accident if you stay there a moment longer. So you carefully edge out of harm's way, no decision having been made.

Action What are you avoiding by making no choices? Understand that the more you procrastinate, the more you are likely to get harmed—by other people's angry frustration. Think before you wander into situations unprepared. Be clear on how to act so that everyone may move forward.

NIGHTMARE CROSSROADS

In the dream, you are living at busy crossroads. Traffic lights flash all night, the noise of vehicles stopping and starting is incessant below your window, and thin curtains let in the cars' bright headlights. Sleep is impossible, and you feel a sense of deep despair.

Action Acknowledge that your life seems to have sunk into a sad place. Accept things could and will get better, but in the meantime, learn to put up with unpleasant conditions, whatever they are.

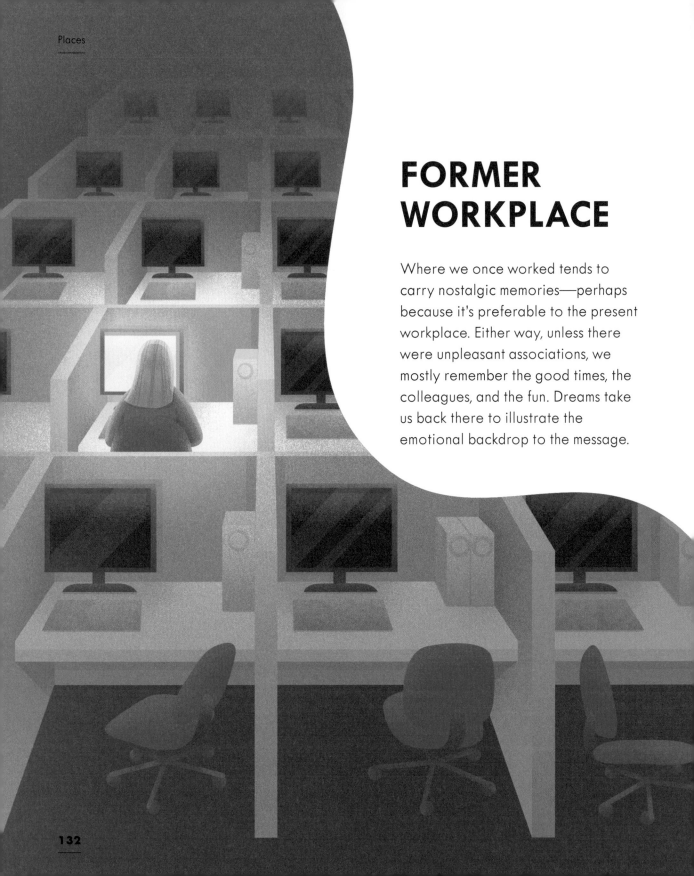

FORMER WORKPLACE

Where we once worked tends to carry nostalgic memories—perhaps because it's preferable to the present workplace. Either way, unless there were unpleasant associations, we mostly remember the good times, the colleagues, and the fun. Dreams take us back there to illustrate the emotional backdrop to the message.

LOVERS AT A FORMER WORKPLACE

You and your lover are ballroom dancing in a former workplace. Waltzing between the work areas, you are watched by admiring colleagues who are amazed by your style and grace. Suddenly everyone disappears, and you are left on your own. It seems all wrong, and you wake feeling dismayed.

Action Things are off kilter; your present relationship may be only half-nourished by your turning psychologically to old pleasures and places. You might not be aware of this or appreciate the need to grow into a new way of relating. If the current relationship is to thrive, don't look back.

THE WORKPLACE IS DERELICT

Seated across from you at their desk is a former colleague. The office is otherwise deserted, no other furniture but for the two desks and computers, and it looks as if the workplace will soon be torn down. What's happened? You ask your colleague, but they don't know the answer. You feel like a ghost in a ghostly office.

Action Is this dream about an office you worked in years ago? Are you nostalgic for those old times, when there was plenty of fun activity and enjoyable work to do? Though it's not possible to recreate what is gone, it is possible to look for new interests—or employment—in the future. Accept the past is past, a first step toward greater fulfillment.

YOU'RE BACK AT YOUR OLD DESK

Back in a former workplace, you are sitting at your desk feeling nostalgic. You long for your old colleagues and friends—perhaps a lover?—and wander down the office aisles, wishing you were still working there. But nobody is recognizing you. It's as if you'd never been with them.

Action You have to accept that you might have made a mistake by leaving that employment. Of course, you may be accepted back again on application, but if this isn't possible, move on. Try ruminating on your hasty decision-making. You could find this propensity needs reining in.

YOUR COWORKERS IGNORE YOU

You're back at work as normal, but your colleagues look different from how you remember them. They are talking sweetly to one another but not to you, and you feel ill at ease. You want to ask them why they are behaving so casually—but no one seems to understand what you mean, and they act as if nothing has changed.

Action Your coworkers may not have been the kindest people. Accept that they jeopardized your integrity daily in subtle ways. Soon, it may seem timely that you left. You are wiser now and can find more authentic places in which you make real friends.

AN UNKNOWN LANDSCAPE

An unfamiliar landscape is territory we have yet to discover. Before the wetlands in America were charted, they were unknown; before man went to the moon, the reality of its surface was unknown. We dream of landscapes unfamiliar to us for a reason—our psyche, in framing a dream scenario against the backdrop of an unknown setting, is sending us a message.

AN EMPTY VILLAGE

Schools, cottages, and the streets are all empty. It feels uncanny and certainly desolate. You peek in some of the cottage windows—no sign of life, just trash, as if the owners left in a hurry and hadn't bothered cleaning up. The village has been abandoned. You feel as desolate as its streets.

Action Is there some part of you that is all alone and feeling abandoned? The metaphor of an empty village in your dream illustrates how you currently see your real-life situation. If you are tied to a daily routine and need more companionship or emotional nourishment, consider how best to find it.

LOST IN AN UNKNOWN LANDSCAPE

You are lost in a landscape you don't recognize. Although you have a map and compass, you find it impossible to read it or make any sense of your bearings. There are other walkers far off; you hurry to join them to ask where you are, but no one can understand what you're saying.

Action An aspect of you is lost. You have a plan—the equivalent of the dream's map—but you aren't putting it into operation. What's stopping you? Learn how to communicate more clearly with those around you and watch how this helps you find out where you are in life and which direction to take.

A RIDE INTO THE UNKNOWN

A driver has stopped to give you a ride. You left the outskirts of a town and realize you are traveling unexpectedly through wild countryside. Alarmed, you see the landscape is unrecognizable. Your driver appears increasingly sinister looking as he pulls his vehicle onto the shoulder: now you fear the worst. But he has only lost his way! His satellite navigation misdirected him to this unknown landscape. You pull out your own map and show him the right route.

Action This dream shows how easy it is to jump to the wrong conclusions. Whenever you consider your situation only, realize occasionally other people might be struggling with their own worries. Try looking at all viewpoints before you make snap decisions: your psyche shows you have the resources to help them.

A CITY LANDSCAPE

City workers are pouring out of offices, making their way toward some unknown place. You follow them. But the city landscape you see after a while is not to your liking. You wish you hadn't followed these people without thinking: you end up lost down a dirty alley.

Action It's time to think for yourself and use your own judgment—not other peoples'.

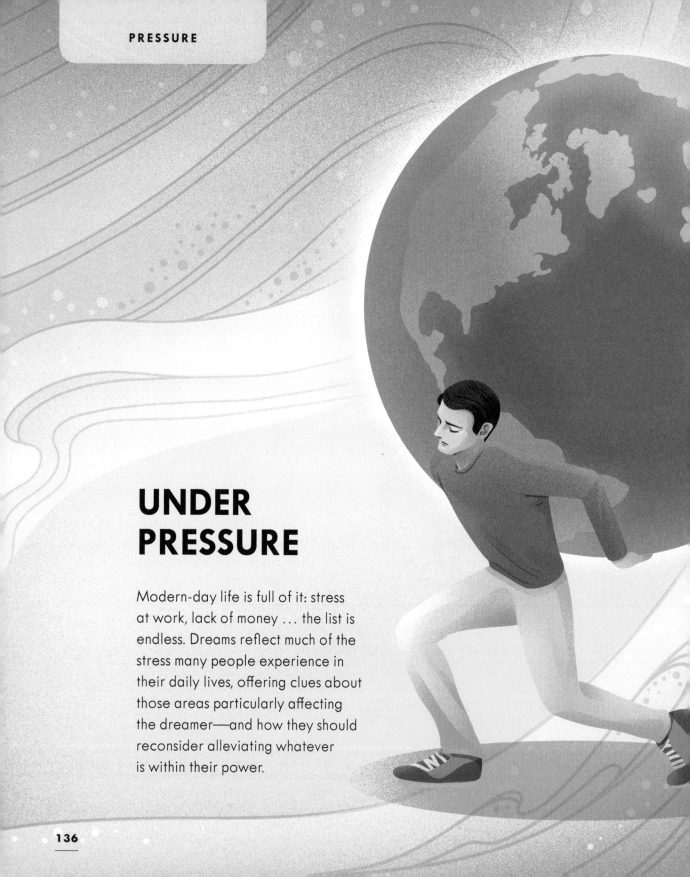

UNDER PRESSURE

Modern-day life is full of it: stress at work, lack of money … the list is endless. Dreams reflect much of the stress many people experience in their daily lives, offering clues about those areas particularly affecting the dreamer—and how they should reconsider alleviating whatever is within their power.

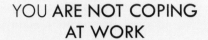

YOU ARE NOT COPING AT WORK

The pressure of work is driving you to take desperate measures. You cut corners, miss urgent appointments, and arrive at those you do keep dressed in your pajamas. Your boss wants to see you to review your work, and you know you will be fired if you haven't secured more deals. You wake up shaking with fear.

Action This driven schedule must stop! Weigh the pros and cons of your situation—perhaps an overfilled home life is indirectly portrayed in the dream?—and carefully mull over that mental list. You are overwhelmed with the pressure upon you. Find ways to ease the burden.

A GLOBE ON YOUR SHOULDERS

A toy globe is perched on your shoulders in the dream, and you stagger under its weight. You hear someone moaning in misery, and you face another day of looking after them, as well as a dozen other responsibilities. There's no escape from this burden, and you long to throw the globe away. But it stays firmly in place.

Action Reflect on how much you are actually carrying in your daily life. You may not appreciate the enormity of the load you're bearing—or realize that it needs readjustment. Plan ways you can lessen the metaphorical weight on your shoulders.

YOUR OFFICE DESK IS PILED HIGH

You watch a pile of paperwork on your desk growing higher and higher. You can't reach the top of it, standing on your tiptoes to try to pull down a handful so that you can get on with your work. You feel desperately trapped—if you don't get through this pile, others will suffer.

Action Talk to whoever has given you this work and explain that you are exhausted. Don't be afraid of letting people down—it would be so much worse if you had to stop due to illness from fatigue. Expect sympathetic understanding, or assert yourself to get it.

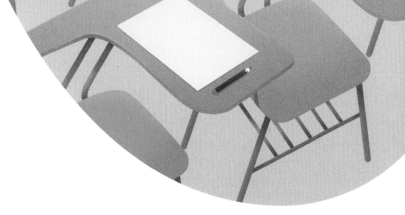

TESTS AND EXAMS

If we dream of taking a test or exam, it usually carries threads of anxiety—unless we enjoy easily acquired achievement. But what if a test isn't to assess our ability, but a medical one over which we have no control? Anxiety is more likely then to trickle into our dream world.

YOU FAIL A MEDICAL EXAM

The doctor examines you during a check-up and insists you have multiple problems, adamant you will be healed as soon as you change your lifestyle. Yet you know you are healthy and angrily demand the doctor rethink the diagnosis. Your insistence is refused.

Action Is this a denial dream? As the doctor, you know your body might benefit from a lifestyle change and that your habits could seriously undermine your long-term health. But as the patient, you are conflicted about giving up so much. Talk with your two parts and listen carefully to the wiser one.

YOUR TEST PAPERS MAKE NO SENSE

You are in an testing room, other candidates busily scribbling their answers to the questions. Yours make no sense; the words or calculations are gobbledegook, and you throw your pen down on the desk and walk out, exasperated.

Action If you are contemplating studying for a career or retraining, consider that it may not be right for you. Have you thought it all through? Even if glittering prizes await, are you really equipped to tackle getting to that level? There's no shame in changing your plans. In the dream, remember you walked out, exasperated: a helpful warning?

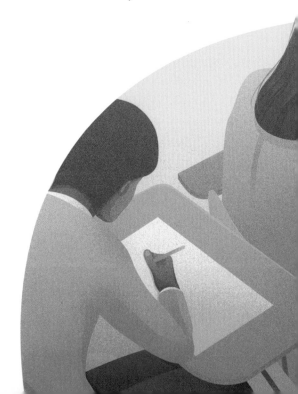

TAKING **YOUR DRIVER'S TEST**

You are a learner driver taking your first driver's test. The car stalls at traffic lights. Embarrassed, you try to start up the engine again, but the car just won't get into action. Despite the turmoil you feel, aware of the examiner quietly sitting beside you, you look in the rearview mirror and see the drivers behind waiting patiently. They're not honking. It's as if they understand what you're going through.

Action You are being tested on something you're engaged in currently and expect people around you to be less than kind. This is your fear, rather than the reality. Decide to change your attitude—try expecting them to be tolerant of your mistakes. You could be surprised by how sympathetic they are.

YOU **ARE UNPREPARED FOR A TEST**

Uneasily, you walk into the students' testing room and sit down at your desk. The question papers, turned facedown, fill you with dread. When it is time to turn them over and start writing, you realize you are totally unprepared. There is next to nothing you can think of to write down, and your heart sinks. What will your family say?

Action Not only were you unprepared for this dream test, you don't appear to want to take it. Who are you trying to please? It's certainly not yourself, or you would have done the necessary work to pass. Resolve to stop trying to meet others' expectations and hopes, and instead follow your own wishes.

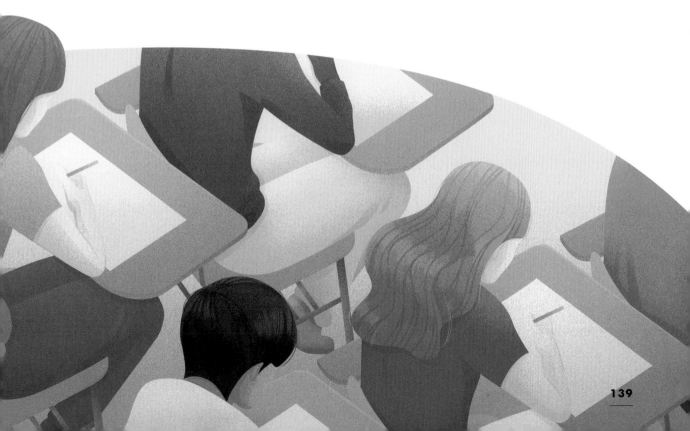

BEING CHASED

There's something primeval about the concept of being chased, whether by an animal or a person. Both could be dangerous and possibly kill you. On the other hand, either could chase you around the garden—or the bedroom—in a fun game without any fear of catastrophe. The dream context will indicate friend or foe.

WILD **ANIMAL CLAWING AT THE DOOR**

A huge wild animal is chasing you out of the woods. Terrified, you run for safety. You peer from a wayside hut's front door and see it coming closer. You slam the door, then hear scratching claws on the woodwork.

Action This wild animal is no marauding monster. He's your dream ally, wanting to help. Find the courage to dream the dream on and invite him inside. Imagine what your ally is trying to convey. Does he want to support in some way, psychologically empowering you? Consider a large wild animal's strength: could you do with some of that?

DANGER **ZONE WARNING**

A man starts to shout from afar and chase you across a field. You start to run in the dream, not liking the look of him and feeling frightened. The yells then inexplicably stop. Suddenly, a barbed-wire fence stretches across the plain in front of you, not far from army huts. So the shouting was a warning—you've wandered into a military zone.

Action Preconceptions can cloud issues, as this dream shows. Try living more authentically, without making false assumptions based on how people look. Learn to wait to find out about them—never assume.

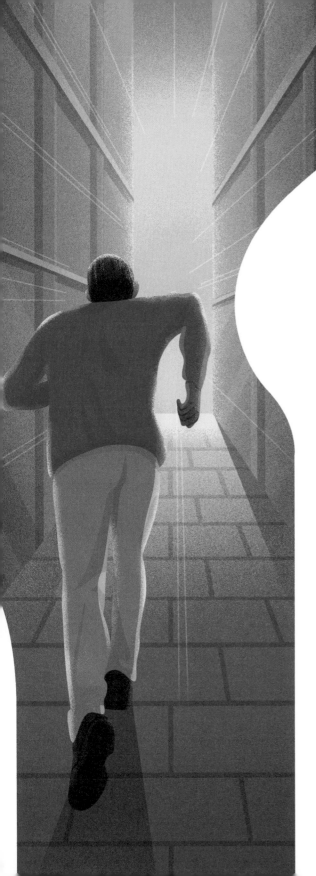

CHASED **BY YOUR PET**

Your pet is curled up fast asleep. There's something you want to make him do, so you wake him. He's frustrated at being disturbed. He leaps growling out of the chair, then chases you around the house. You try to pacify him, but the damage is done: he'll be touchy all day.

Action Who might the animal be representing—someone you know, or a part of yourself longing to just curl up and shut out the world? Either way, appreciate how an abrupt wakening is upsetting—and you must pay the consequences. Try easing gently into situations, for another's sake or for your own.

FOOTSTEPS **FOLLOW YOU DOWN A DARK STREET**

You are hurrying home from an evening out and hear footsteps behind you. The quicker you walk, the faster the steps become: someone is chasing you and means you harm! You start to run—so does the follower. Frightened, you aim for a stranger's front door. Your pursuer catches up to you, but they hurry past. You feel foolish.

Action Fear makes us imagine the worst. Are you often anxious, identifying with the plight of assaulted victims you read about? You are not alone in struggling with fear: no need to feel foolish. Own your fears by sharing your feelings with a good friend—then those scary dreams may be less likely to return.

BEING LATE

Being late for an appointment is usually a source of great pressure. Dreams often feature that frantic need to meet a deadline of some sort and reflect the dreamer's anxiety about failing to be dependable—socially, professionally, or in relationships. These dreams can be useful in helping us learn more about ourselves in order to face those challenges.

YOU **ARE LATE** FOR A FUNERAL

You have to speak at a funeral and the deceased relatives will be waiting for you, but you are stuck in traffic. There is no chance of reaching the cemetary in time. It's impossible to turn around; you turn off the engine and wait, desolate to be letting down the mourners.

Action The dream indicates you could feel a bit overly responsible for others' feelings. If it's impossible to keep an appointment—distressing them through no fault of your own—then it's important to learn you can't always get it right, even though you like pleasing people.

YOU **ARE LATE FOR** SCHOOL PICK-UP

You are due to pick up a child from school, so you finish some work, then hurry as fast as you can to the school grounds. All of the children have gone home with their caregivers—only the child you are collecting is left, weeping bitterly. You feel remorseful but helpless in the face of such a busy working afternoon.

Action This dream is a warning about not taking on any task you're in danger of failing to carry through. Consider how to rearrange your routine to cope with the unexpected, and learn to say no when it's appropriate.

YOU **ARE LATE FOR** YOUR OWN WEDDING

Guests and your future marriage partner are waiting for you. Dressed for your wedding, you discover your feet inexplicably will not move from the bedroom: you are stuck to the floor. You simply cannot leave and walk downstairs. Not only will you be late, it clearly looks as if you won't be making it to the wedding at all.

Action The wedding is a metaphor for a major life decision. This dream is about being caught in a conflicting state of mind, with part of you wanting to move on and part of you not. This ambiguity can in fact bring about an emotional paralysis. Listen to your frightened part, try talking to it, and understand anxiety is probably what's holding you back.

FALLING

Few dreamers have not experienced that uncomfortable feeling of dropping through the air, falling like a stone. Falling is associated with not being in charge, and such negativity tends to collect bad vibes. Even falling in love carries some negative connotations, usually because it means we're out of control again.

YOU ARE FALLING INTO WATER

You are swimming in fast-running water with a group of friends. Suddenly you are swept up in the current and plunged over a drop to fall into swirling waters below. Everyone is safe: there's nothing to do but go with the current.

Action Is there a parallel here with your daily life? If all you can do is go with the flow, embrace the conditions and see where the flow takes you. Safety lies ahead—and you may even enjoy getting there.

FALLING FROM A HEIGHT

You dream of climbing a steep hill so you can admire the view. It is superb, and you lean forward to see better around a corner—but you overbalance and find yourself falling a long way to the ground. When you jolt awake, you are more than thankful to be safe in bed.

Action So you overstretched yourself enjoying the view, but this dream actually shows you taking stock of your life's panorama so far. Foolhardy maybe, but take comfort in the fact that you had the strength to climb that hill to get to this viewpoint. Remember to be extra careful now that you have reached this breadth of psychological vision. The words "pride" and "fall" should come to mind.

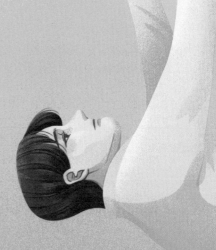

YOUR **PARACHUTE** WON'T OPEN

The moment has come for your parachute jump. Your instructor yells for you to prepare, and at his command, you jump. Falling fast through the air, you guess that it's time to open the chute, but it fails to deploy. As you hurtle toward a certain death, you tug once more on the resistant release device. The canopy finally billows out—you're saved!

Action Taking risks with proper preparation is one thing; doing the same with an unreliable fallback is another. Remember, you need to surround yourself with experts, take advice from the professionals, and not undertake dangerous enterprises—including emotional ones—without care.

YOU **WATCH A CHILD FALL**

Out in the park, you watch children climbing trees and remember the fun you had as a child. You then notice one boy negotiating a dead branch halfway up the tree and idly wonder what will happen next. The branch snaps, releasing the climber just as an adult passerby runs to break his fall. They both end up unhurt, laughing on the ground. You wish you'd thought quickly enough, too.

Action Watching a childhood adventure is, of course, pleasurable for the good memories it evokes and vicarious enjoyment. But you have a responsibility to safeguard little kids in potentially dangerous situations. If you're a parent, remember a child takes risks to learn—be ever watchful.

SQUEEZING THROUGH A HOLE

There's no avoiding the obvious scenario that comes to mind—a baby being born—but of course there are many other ways our dreams can infer birth of another kind. They can depict a new chapter, transition, or difficult maneuvers. But central to all images of squeezing through tight spaces is the concept of change.

AN ENTRANCE IS TOO NARROW

A storm is brewing, and you hurry to find shelter from the rain. You see an old hut as the rain begins to pour down, and you rush toward it. The hut's door is only half-open, and you try to squeeze through the small space. But it's impossible. You have a growing fear that you're stuck, unable to go forward or backward.

Action The storm—whatever this represents—has pushed you into a situation you may not yet be ready for. Resign yourself to waiting for matters to subside and hope that next time you will be able to make the difficult journey through that narrow entrance.

YOU ARE STUCK IN A MANHOLE IN THE ROAD

Torrential rain has caused severe flooding. A manhole outside has been lifted by the torrent underground, and you think it is your job to get it sorted out. You climb down but somehow get stuck. You wish you'd called others to help before venturing down there on your own.

Action Reflect how much you rush in to take on jobs for which you are not prepared. Enlist expert help before you undertake risky projects. You can achieve far more together.

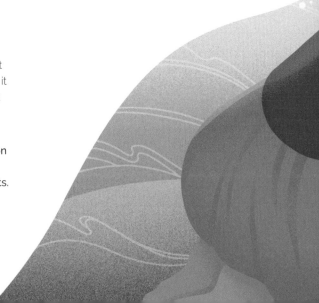

YOU WITNESS A DIFFICULT HOSPITAL BIRTH

A woman is in labor, and you watch her struggle to give birth to her baby. The attending doctor and nurses seem to be getting anxious. There is talk of a cesarean section, and you know the woman is distressed. You are concerned, but mostly for her unborn infant, with whom you feel closely linked.

Action In this dream, you are the fetus, trying in the outer world to squeeze through blockages holding you back from experiencing a new life for yourself. Try to relax and wait patiently. You succeeded once—now your birth is symbolic, preparing to free you for happier times ahead.

YOU HAVE GROWN TOO LARGE TO FIT

At work in your usual office, you suddenly realize you have grown enormous. Everyone else is their normal size, but you are huge by comparison. You want to speak to your employer and go toward their door. No one notices your disproportionate size except you, because it's impossible to squeeze through the open office door.

Action This dream may be indicating you have outgrown your present work or place of employment. Are you ready for more of a challenge? It could be time to plan a new career elsewhere—somewhere you'll fit in with like-minded people at the same intellectual level.

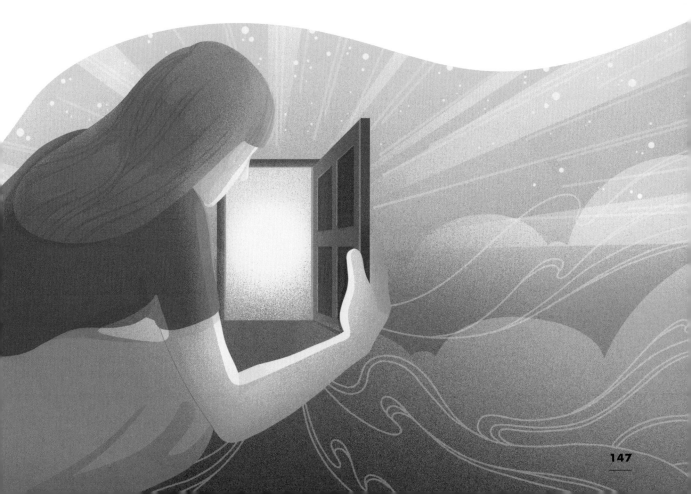

MARATHON RUNNING

Dreams of extreme physical endurance offer glimpses into the dreamer's unconscious view of themselves—resilient or lightweight?—or perhaps wishful thinking about applause and glory. They hint, too, at darker material: of endurance and effort.

YOU ARE WEARING THE WRONG SHOES

You discover you're wearing the wrong shoes for the terrain as you take part in a mountain marathon with dozens of other runners. The shoes begin to disintegrate, but in the dream, you're not bothered about competing anyway. By now barefoot, you can still run comfortably, enjoying the view. You reach the finish line to sympathetic applause, the last competitor.

Action Unlike the successful runners, you enjoyed the view instead of seriously competing. What does the dream marathon symbolize? Do you have what it takes to agree to a big commitment? Though you are not well equipped, are you still capable of finishing the course and even enjoying the enterprise?

A WORK MARATHON

Your workload reaches nightmare proportions as you are required to do far more than you can cope with. You're asked to make difficult calls, write a thousand words, pick up the children from school, prepare for a dinner party ... You're in despair at this "running around" and feel so resentful, you punch the nearest person hard.

Action Passive aggression lurks here in real life! Think about how often you let others put upon you, probably unaware of the difficulty they cause. Voice your concerns before you take it out on the perpetrators, as you did in the dream. Find the courage to explain your feelings about being overloaded. Express your anger for a change; others will be glad you did, despite your usual diffidence.

A SNOWBOUND RACE

You have prepared for weeks to run in a charity race, but one glance outside shows the streets are snowbound. You wish you hadn't enrolled—all those wasted hours training when you needed to do other things. But your dream takes you to the starting line, and only a handful of runners have turned up. You all decide to carry on, trudging companionably through the snow.

Action Celebrate your determination. That attitude to continue on despite setbacks is a gift to be proud of, whether it's a marathon or facing life's inevitable challenges.

YOU STRUGGLE TO REACH THE FINISH LINE

Runners are passing you in the dream's race, and although you can see the finish line, you just cannot reach it. Now you are crawling, exhausted, as the crowds dwindle away, the race over. But a friend appears and helps you get to your feet again and stagger to the end.

Action Learn to look after yourself better. Are you setting unrealistic goals, not fully prepared? Realize how much better you'd feel if you had trained—whatever training means for you—and continue to the end, confident the long distance ahead is possible.

> "FIVE MINUTES ARE ENOUGH TO DREAM A WHOLE LIFE, THAT IS HOW RELATIVE TIME IS."

MARIO BENEDETTI

WORK PERFORMANCE

Nowadays, the pressure of giving a good performance has never been so foremost in people's minds. Whatever the setting, delivering at work appears to be key to a promotion, or to getting fired if you're not up to the task. Dreams reflect this current anxiety, sometimes focusing on the unexpected.

YOU'RE APPLAUDED FOR YOUR WORK

In your dream, you watch two nurses frantically performing resuscitation on a patient in cardiac arrest. One of them is you. The patient suddenly recovers, sits up in bed, and beams their gratitude. The watching hospital staff applaud the two nurses, who take a bow.

Action As one of the nurses, you are being reassured that you're doing an excellent job in your own situation. Be proud of your expertise and dedication to the work you chose—whatever its real setting—but be sure to sign up for continuing professional development or similar nurturing activities.

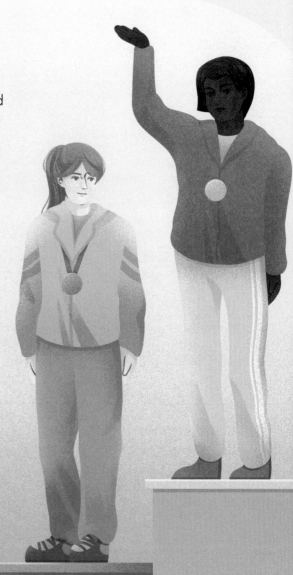

YOU **LOSE CONCENTRATION**

Part of a workforce, you are a bricklayer building a block of apartments. It's monotonous, and you begin making pretty patterns with the bricks. So absorbed in this, you fail to notice water seeping through the holes left by your artistry. Too late, you realize the building's safety could be compromised by your thoughtlessness.

Action Examine your daytime behavior. Are you paying too much attention to trivial stuff? Take this dream as a warning: creativity is good, but not if you jeopardize the structure of your work and home life.

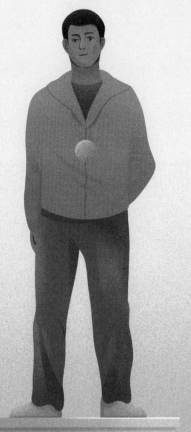

YOU **ARE TOLD YOUR WORK IS NOT GOOD ENOUGH**

Your manager tells you that your performance is not up to snuff. You are amazed—you imagined everyone was delighted with your work. The manager implies that if you can't deliver better in the future, you're fired. A colleague then appears and offers to show you how to meet the company's expectations.

Action Have you been too casual about your work performance in reality? Accept that there is a divide between their expectations and your own, despite your belief all was well. The colleague is a part of yourself; learn to follow your own innate wisdom.

THE **WORKERS ARE INEPT**

Farm workers are guiding a herd of animals down a street. At first, you see them in control of the pigs and cows, but when the farmers start to wave their sticks around helplessly, you are shocked at their ineptitude. Some animals have broken into nearby stores and are creating havoc. You blame the farm workers for failing to control them.

Action Here, you are being given a two-pronged message. You are both the group of animals creating havoc and the inept farm hands. Are you guilty of running wild (the animals) and making foolish decisions (the workers)? Others may notice and judge your work performance accordingly if you fail to resolve that inner conflict.

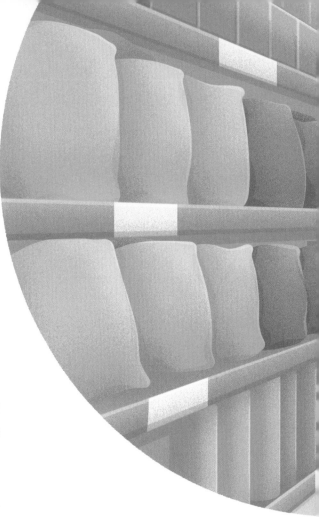

NAKED IN PUBLIC

Ask anyone the most embarrassing situation they fear most and the answer would probably involve being seen naked in public. However, to be seen without your clothes on can also be a liberating experience. Dreams of public nudity can be revealing in more ways than one, mirroring anxiety or reflecting an inner confidence.

YOU **ARE NAKED ONSTAGE**

You walk onstage to give a talk. You can't understand why members of the audience begin to whisper behind their hands and why some are even laughing. You then realize to your shame that you are completely naked. However, you continue your talk, and when it comes to its natural conclusion, the audience claps enthusiastically. You are congratulated later for the speech—not for your courage.

Action Take heart from this dream. Instead of rushing offstage, you found the courage to carry on. Your authenticity is clear: the audience was compelled to listen to your talk, not snicker at your nudity. Take this awareness into your daily life—it will serve you well.

YOU **ARE NAKED IN A SWIMMING POOL**

You are diving into a pool with many others, all wearing swimming gear. Before surfacing, you notice they are naked, and so are you. But when you next see them, they are dressed as usual. You remain naked, completely at ease.

Action Water in this dream represents the world of the unconscious: most people are not yet ready to peel off their protective layers, and you cannot speed them toward the same state you have reached. Be glad you have achieved an inner balance between conscious and unconscious—its hidden depths hold no fear for you.

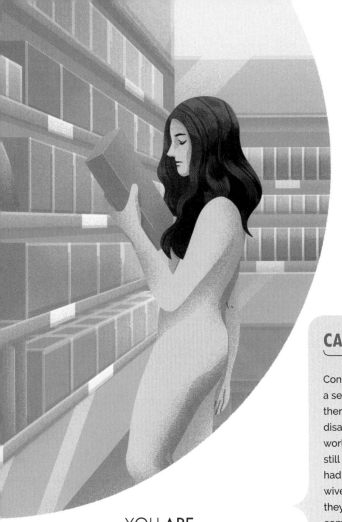

YOU **ARE** SHOPPING NAKED

You find yourself walking out of a store naked onto a crowded street. Unconcerned, you wander down the street to look into other windows. The reflection of you naked, surrounded by stunned crowds, does not embarrass you. You like what you see, warts and all, and enjoy how unencumbered you feel.

Action Your dream mirrors an inner confidence. Be proud to be seen, even if this cannot in reality mean being unclothed in public. Understand you have reached a stage in your psychological development where you feel no need to hide your true self, complete with imperfections.

CASE STUDY: CONNOR

Connor was the older son of a strict father and a selfish mother. He did his best to please them, learning to hide his anger and disappointment behind gentle compliance. It worked for everyone. Middle-aged, he was still running his survival script. Two marriages had failed to show him what was wrong. His wives didn't like him going for solitary walks; they complained that he was uncomfortably compliant yet selfish in his lack of consideration. Connor then had a revelation.

He dreamed he was at home plate in a baseball game, waiting completely naked and unconcerned—illustrating his nonawareness—for the next pitch. The ball hit him on his forehead and knocked him sideways. He heard the words "Now will you get it, dumbo?", as if the carefully aimed pitch was designed to knock some sense into his head. The dream message hit home.

He invited his next girlfriend to join him on his walks; he stopped being too agreeable; and sometimes, when appropriate, he gets really angry. They are doing just fine.

MISSING BODY PARTS

The idea of losing any part of our body holds primitive fear: at a base level, we believe a missing limb—or whatever part it may be—means we are less able to survive. Of course, we can and we do, but the loss usually represents a sense of powerlessness.

YOUR **ARMS HAVE BEEN SEVERED**

You wake from an anesthetic and remember why you're in a hospital bed. Your arms have been cut off. The horror increases when you realize it's not even possible to feel where and how: you have no hands to search, and the feeling of powerlessness is overwhelming. You scream out, but no one answers.

Action Consider the reason for such a harrowing dream. It's likely to be based on recent events, where you felt either unable to lash out verbally or blamed yourself for having such powerful physical feelings against someone. Your psyche played out the damage for you. Now you must contemplate how better to resolve the problem. If talking doesn't work, try piling up cushions and punching them— in the privacy of your bedroom.

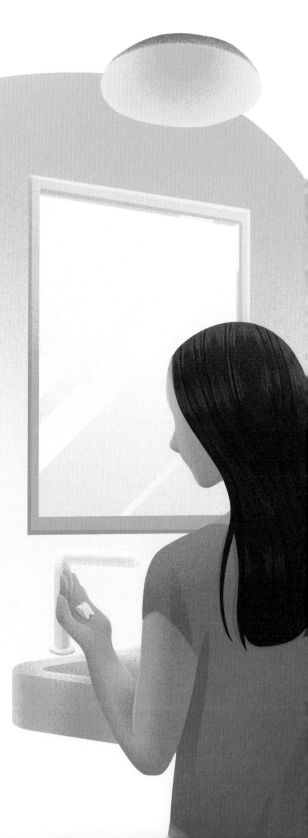

YOU CUT OFF YOUR HAIR

Staying overnight with a group of strangers where everyone shares dormitory rooms, you notice one person takes off a wig to reveal a bald head. Devastated at this shocking hair loss, you pick up some scissors and cut off chunks of your own hair to show your sympathy.

Action You have empathy for others, as this dream shows. But there's more: you are also the bald person, taking off a wig to sleep. Are you afraid of losing your hair—if not fully, maybe with a daring new style—and you fear others' reactions? The scissors gesture appeared kind, but it gave an equivocal message. As the bald person, would witnessing it really have helped your own situation? Consider the lesson here.

YOUR TEETH ARE FALLING OUT

As you brush your teeth, you watch horrified as some of them clatter into the sink. You pick them up and try to glue them back into your gums, but they fall out again and again.

Action Ask yourself what's going on that feels difficult to chew on or bite through. If a major decision is the issue, you may need to reflect carefully on the best options. If there's potentially a high cost at risk—emotionally or financially—this may have presented your unconscious with a warning. Write down all of the pros and cons and see if deliberating firmly on them will help steer you away from biting off more than you can chew.

CASE STUDY: CAMERON

Cameron had been a rugby player and keen golfer. One day, out of the blue, he suffered a serious stroke and lost the use of his right arm. Walking was difficult, as his right leg was affected, too, but he managed to work toward some kind of rehabilitation.

The loss of the use in his right arm affected him deeply. He could no longer write, drive a car, or play golf—and consequently lost most of his old social contacts. As a result, he sank into depression.

He then had a dream. He was shown a review of his long life—brave war pilot, father to five loving children from two long marriages (he'd been widowed in midlife), and busy school teacher. But in the dream, he was paralyzed! "Watching" his autobiographical narrative, he was aware that he was unable to move, experiencing the full horror of total immobility. When he woke, Cameron realized he'd lost nothing but the use of his arm, compared to what might have been. The dream helped him reappraise his situation and eased him into acceptance.

LOST WALLET

A wallet or purse holds not only
our money and credit cards, but
also our driver's license, membership
cards, and often private treasures.
When it goes missing, it's as if our
identity has been stolen: the loss
carries psychological implications.
When we dream of losing our wallet
or purse, we dream of the fear of
losing a part of ourselves.

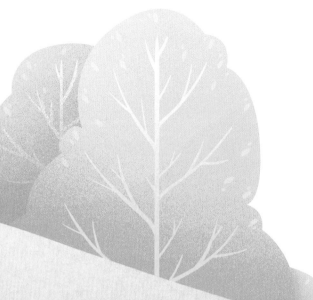

YOUR **WALLET GOES MISSING ON A JOURNEY**

In the middle of a train journey to a new destination, you are asked to show your ticket. You reach for your wallet; it is missing. You search among your pockets, but it is nowhere to be found—no ticket, no money. Frightened, you wake up with a jolt.

Action You want to explore new places and yearn for a break. But your dream indicates you haven't thought through the details closely enough. If a change is planned, pay attention to your finances. Your "ticket" also represents the practicalities involved in making changes. Is it appropriate to consider them right now?

YOU **TRY TO BUY FRIENDSHIP**

In a strange town, you're at the bar about to buy a lonely drink. A large group of people arrive and start to order their drinks. Anxious in the dream to make friends quickly and be popular, you offer to pay for a round. When the bartender tells you how much you owe, you reach for your wallet and are shocked: it's no longer there. Everyone picks up their chosen drink and carries on talking among themselves, ignoring you.

Action Buying friendship in real life doesn't work. Those people had their own agendas to make friends and be popular. No one in your dream noticed your predicament, nor did anyone offer to pay your bar tab. Surely, the first step to a real friendship might mean waiting for the authentic ones to come to you first, or you offering to help them out of a difficult situation, like the dream scenario.

YOU **CAN'T PAY FOR YOUR ITEMS**

You are on a spending spree, selecting only expensive items. At the register, your goods are packed; laden plastic bags sit on the counter. The time has arrived to pay, but your wallet, containing all your money and cards, is missing. Mortified, you watch the assistants take the bags away. They look embarrassed.

Action What events led up to this dream? Are you aching to spend money you don't have? On one level, the dream offers you the goods you think you want—but is that really true? On another level, there's a high price to pay, and your psyche has shown you embarrassment all around if you decide to embark on a spending spree. Be patient and wait to save up money only for what you can afford.

"

I DREAM OF
PAINTING AND THEN
I PAINT MY DREAM.

"

VINCENT VAN GOGH
THE LETTERS OF VINCENT VAN GOGH

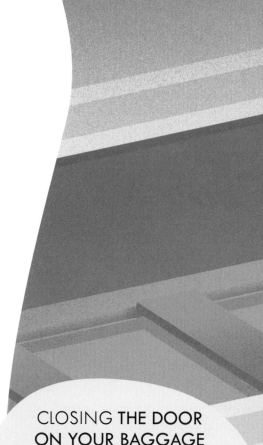

BAGGAGE LEFT BEHIND

Leaving baggage behind is an uncomfortable situation. It could mean retracing our steps, spending money on important items that we already own in order to go forward. But dreams of this nature can also carry a positive twist: we speak of "baggage" when we refer to neuroses. So if it's left behind, that can only be good news.

CLOSING THE DOOR ON YOUR BAGGAGE

In this dream, you see yourself shutting the front door of a house for what you know will be the last time. Your problems have been resolved; your worrying and obsessing are neuroses of the past. You have left your emotional baggage behind in that house.

Action This kind of dream applies to many of life's decisions—ending a relationship, leaving home, finishing therapy—but knowing when it is time to go it alone is an important stage in your development. Be thankful for the opportunity learned to strike out on your own and pat yourself on the back.

YOU LEAVE YOUR SUITCASE ON THE PLATFORM

As your train pulls out of the station, you realize you've left your suitcase behind on the platform. It holds your dressiest clothes and the only copy of a speech you have to make on arrival. Instead of panicking, you shrug, order a cup of coffee, and relax.

Action You have learned how to accept whatever life throws at you. You know your impromptu speech will go well and that appearance is unimportant. Celebrate the dream's confirmation that it's wisdom and experience that counts.

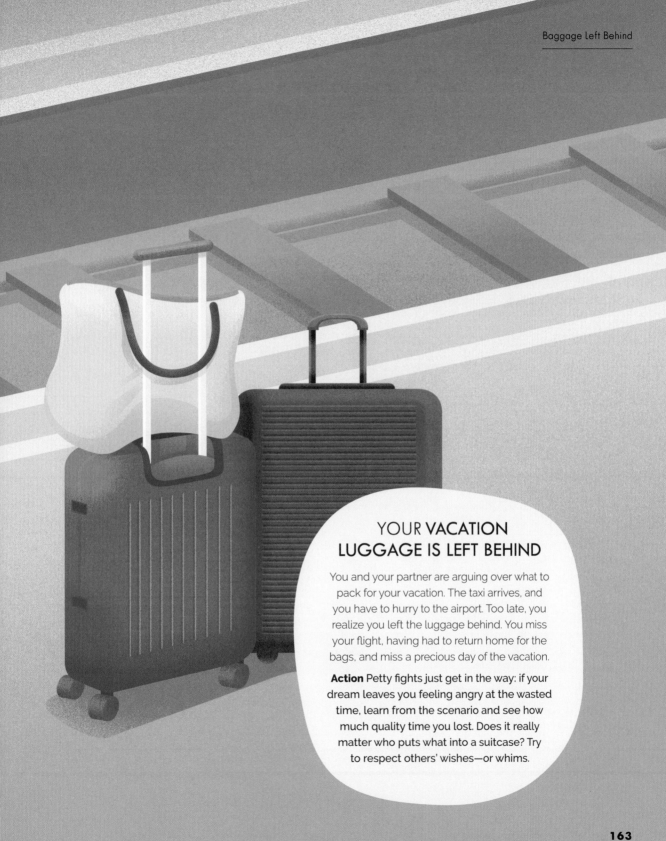

YOUR **VACATION LUGGAGE IS LEFT BEHIND**

You and your partner are arguing over what to pack for your vacation. The taxi arrives, and you have to hurry to the airport. Too late, you realize you left the luggage behind. You miss your flight, having had to return home for the bags, and miss a precious day of the vacation.

Action Petty fights just get in the way: if your dream leaves you feeling angry at the wasted time, learn from the scenario and see how much quality time you lost. Does it really matter who puts what into a suitcase? Try to respect others' wishes—or whims.

REDUNDANCY

Nobody likes being redundant: the word reeks of negativity. We can be made redundant from employment, a team sport, or even a fun outing if the numbers aren't right. It's not always personal; it's usually more about quantity than quality. Yet it always hurts, because the implication is that we're surplus to requirements.

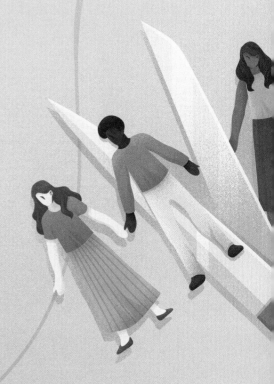

THERE'S A ROBOT AT YOUR DESK

Upon your return to work after a vacation, you find a robot sitting at your desk, doing your job very efficiently. Does this mean you've been made redundant in your absence? You hurry to your manager to hear the confirmation you were dreading.

Action This dream often reflects people's fears when they go on vacation—there are many tales of jobs lost when least expected. Accept that it's about your own fears, maybe fueled by an upcoming vacation, but also wonder if you're keeping up with the times enough. Technology is racing ahead. If you don't want to compete with a robot one day, consider retraining or brushing up on your present skills.

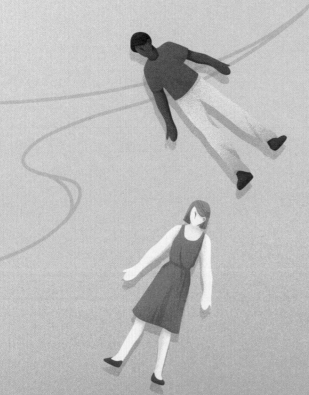

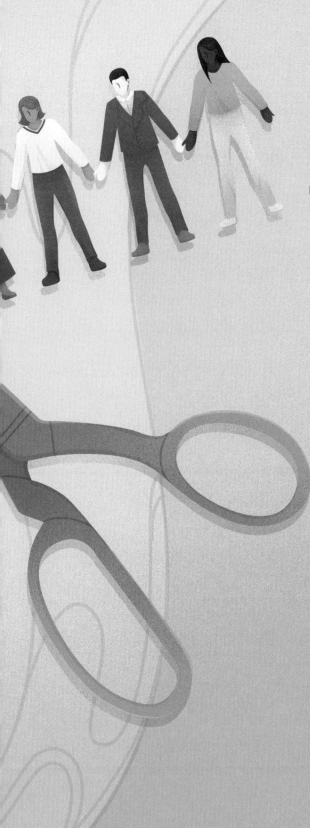

YOU RECEIVE A TERMINATION LETTER

It says it all: "Unfortunately, we are having to let you go ...," and in your dream the world collapses metaphorically around your feet. The shame of losing your job fills you with great embarrassment. Other letters pile up, all demanding payment. You tell yourself that by the end of the month, you'll have nothing to eat.

Action Be thankful it was only a dream—but termination letters or emails do arrive, and we have to accept our fate. Prepare for it by considering how best to arrange your money matters, talk with your family, and plan what changes might have to be made. It may never happen! But this dream is not only about your natural fear of loss or status. Take it as a helpful warning that a layoff can happen to anyone, no matter how skilled. You should feel no shame— see it instead as an unexpected opportunity.

YOU ARE TRYING TO MAKE YOURSELF INDISPENSABLE

Intent on looking after the welfare of your work colleagues, you scurry about in the dream attending to their needs. You're proud of your generosity and enjoy the gratitude they show, but feel surprised your employers haven't commented on your popularity and value. You work more hours than necessary and exhaust yourself with all the effort you put in. Then, suddenly, the bombshell: you've been laid off.

Action Is there a message here about you trying to be indispensable so that you won't be laid off from your job? If the work you're doing in reality is good enough, then any job termination issue would not be about your performance. Cuts have to be made, and another job might one day prove to be a really pleasant change.

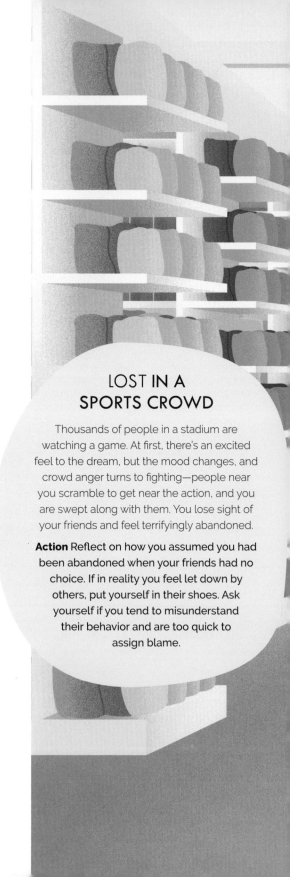

BEING LOST

Dreams relive our deepest fears if they're about being lost somewhere. They echo our primal terror of being alone. Whether the dream setting is a city, forest, or desert, the dread of abandonment is always the same. We see this in waking life, when a newborn baby cries for food. But for an adult, the focus shifts to emotional survival.

LOST IN THE SUPERMARKET

You are a child again, lost in the supermarket and crying in shock. "Where is Mommy? I want my Mommy ...," you call, gazing bewildered down the aisles, feeling certain you've been abandoned. Shoppers nearby try to comfort you, but you know you will never see her again.

Action This is a classic nightmare for a child, but why dream this now? Check to see if there's a close relationship currently in doubt. Understand how deeply childhood dread colors the present, but remember that you and your mother were always reunited, and all was well.

LOST IN A SPORTS CROWD

Thousands of people in a stadium are watching a game. At first, there's an excited feel to the dream, but the mood changes, and crowd anger turns to fighting—people near you scramble to get near the action, and you are swept along with them. You lose sight of your friends and feel terrifyingly abandoned.

Action Reflect on how you assumed you had been abandoned when your friends had no choice. If in reality you feel let down by others, put yourself in their shoes. Ask yourself if you tend to misunderstand their behavior and are too quick to assign blame.

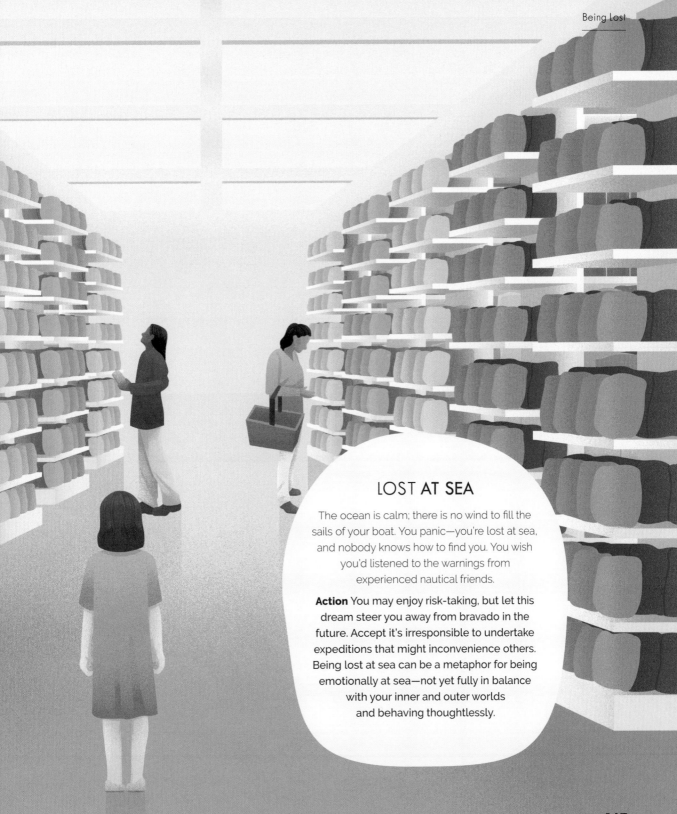

LOST **AT SEA**

The ocean is calm; there is no wind to fill the sails of your boat. You panic—you're lost at sea, and nobody knows how to find you. You wish you'd listened to the warnings from experienced nautical friends.

Action You may enjoy risk-taking, but let this dream steer you away from bravado in the future. Accept it's irresponsible to undertake expeditions that might inconvenience others. Being lost at sea can be a metaphor for being emotionally at sea—not yet fully in balance with your inner and outer worlds and behaving thoughtlessly.

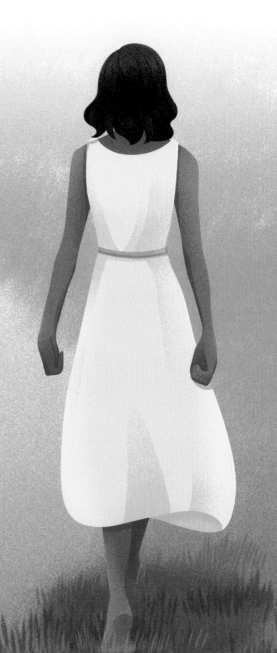

SHOELESS

Being shoeless in dreams can mean pleasant grassy walks in the park or a sandy stroll on the beach. But no footwear might indicate a reluctance to move out into the world. Dreams could highlight an anxiety about facing challenges—an unpreparedness. Though subtle, it could be an unconscious sabotage to avoid going toward something scary out there.

YOU ARE WALKING BAREFOOT

It's a glorious summer's day, and you are walking barefoot in the park. Suddenly, there's an explosion nearby. People run out of the park, away from danger. But you go in the opposite direction, curious to see the damage. You then realize you are shoeless: jagged pieces of metal and burning debris litter the pavement, and you have hurt your feet badly.

Action Is good-turned-bad a frequent theme in your life? Your curiosity led you down the wrong route, and you suffered for it. Consider how to rein in your impetuous actions and learn to be more patient. All will be revealed in due course.

YOU HAVE LOST YOUR SHOES

You have been offered a new job and dream of preparing for Day 1. Should you have had your hair styled? What outfit should you wear, and which shoes? Tension mounts. Where have you put your shoes? You search frantically but find none. Resigned, you take it all as a sign you're meant to stay home.

Action Your dream reflects how daunted you feel about considering taking a new job. It shows you self-sabotaging to stop making any career move. Be glad the dream gave a clear message about your reticence—replace it with courage.

YOU ARE RELUCTANT TO TAKE OFF YOUR SHOES

Upon visiting a temple, your attention is drawn to rows of other people's shoes—sandals, boots, loafers—but you are determined not to take yours off, despite someone's polite request. They might get stolen!

Action Are you too possessive? Is there also a lack of trust here, seldom wanting to risk loss of any sort, even where others are content to trust, as the temple visitors showed? Try not to cling too tightly to your possessions. What is yours will come to you, be it shoes—or perhaps a new relationship.

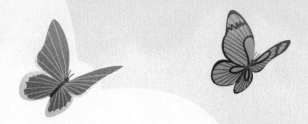
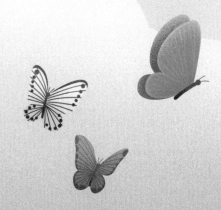

FUNERALS

Usually not a subject to bring light and joy into peoples' lives—quite the opposite, if a loved one has died. But in the dream world, funerals often hold positive messages. While associated, of course, with death and transition, they seldom mean physical death. But change is always indicated.

YOUR OWN FUNERAL

You dream of digging your own grave. You are then killed by a crowd of angry women, who lower you into the ground. They cover you with dirt and prepare to leave you all alone. Somehow you feel a strange sense of rightness, as if these women were justified in their anger and fairly sought to bury you—or was it a part of you?

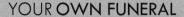

Action This is a symbolic dream, where some ignored aspect of your personality is being taken to task by your psyche. Are you aware of neglecting your feminine, softer, intuitive side? Are you overly proud of your penetrative strength—your masculine power? Man or woman, you should have an equal balance of both masculine and feminine for psychological maturity. Respect the dream's message and work on nurturing your feminine qualities.

A BUTTERFLY AFTER A FUNERAL

Your dream takes you outside into a church's graveyard once the funeral service has finished, and you watch grieving relatives and friends witness the final stages of a loved one's funeral. For you, the loss is deeply felt: you can't imagine life without the presence of that loving person. Suddenly, when the mourners have walked away, you see a butterfly fluttering over the grave.

Action Millions of the world's population believe in life after death. A butterfly is often a symbol of rebirth—it emerges from a chrysalis into a completely new life. Take comfort from the possibility that your dream butterfly is confirming this: it's a beautiful image, and the dream belongs to you.

WATCHING A CELEBRITY'S FUNERAL

In the dream, someone famous has died—a celebrity you have always admired—and you are watching television coverage to share in the mourning. You weep at the first sight of the flower-laden coffin, knowing the person inside is gone forever. Your tears remain as you wake up to reality—and remember they haven't died.

Action This famous person portrays many of the qualities you most wish you possessed yourself. Whatever they are, accept that your grief is not for the dreamed loss of a beloved celebrity, but rather you are grieving for what unconsciously represents the end of hope that you can ever achieve those qualities yourself. You may actually have them but are unaware or lack the confidence to acknowledge their presence. Think about what attracts you to that person. Can you entertain the possibility that you are a bit like them? Practice believing in yourself, and celebrate your own qualities.

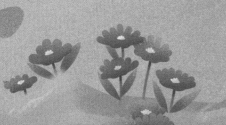

171

DECEASED PETS

The life span of domestic animals is comparatively short, and pets usually die before their owners. Each has a character of their own, giving and receiving affection. Theirs was another heart beating nearby—small wonder we find such pleasure in our pets. We grieve when it's time for them to go, but they often return in our dreams, just when their appearance is most relevant.

A DEAD CANARY'S WARNING

You dream about a dead canary. The pet seems to have died prematurely—had it eaten or breathed something toxic? You go to its cage and gently put the bird into a box, ready to take it outside into the garden.

Action Search for signs of mildew or mold in your home—the spores can become a health hazard. Check the battery in your carbon monoxide alarms, if you have them. Whether it was your deceased pet's warning, or a dream triggered by a news item that day, consider this a potentially useful hint.

YOUR PET IS COMING HOME

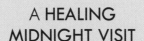

You dream of your pet who died many months ago, high-tailing it home just as she used to do. Overjoyed at the reunion, you open your arms to pick her up to stroke her. But the dream suddenly ends; your beloved companion has left you alone once again.

Action Take comfort from her reappearance. The pain of loss may be hard, but never forget that you had her affection for the time you were together. That cannot die, just as energy cannot die.

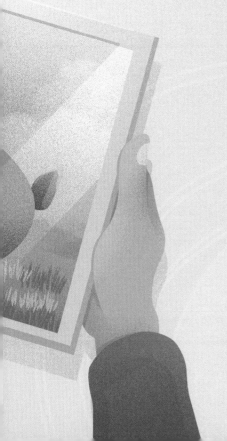

A HEALING MIDNIGHT VISIT

In your dream, you hear scratching at your door at night—it sounds like an animal's request to be let in. You climb out of bed and cautiously open the door. Standing there is a dog you know to be dead in reality. Yet here he is, alive and well.

Action Deceased animals are universally recorded "visiting" people who need healing. Have you been unhappy or unwell? If his appearance cheered you, count it as a healing visit. Be grateful this dog picked up on your needs and somehow checked into your dream world.

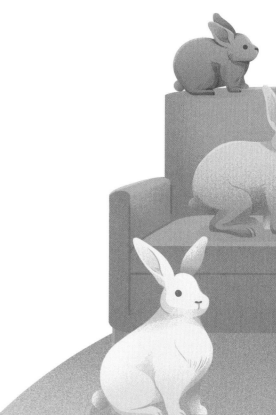

DOMESTIC ANIMALS

Animals in our dreams sometimes represent themselves, or they can indicate an aspect of ourselves. For example, a horse reflects power and sexuality, while a mouse reflects our shyness. Domestic animals were tamed from the wild: we can learn from dreams about them what has been tamed in ourselves—or needs to be.

YOU TRY TO PROTECT YOUR PET

You are going for a walk in the dream with your pet. A loud noise frightens you both, and instinctively you reach out to protect your pet. But the animal—just as instinctively—is frightened for its life and flees in an act of primitive self-protection. You wake regretful that you didn't respect your pet's ability to take care of itself.

Action Instinct overruled precaution here. Bear in mind that a domestic animal carries survival genes despite its adaptation. Can you own the instinctual creature in you—the part not wanting to be protected unnecessarily? Be proud of your independent spirit and don't let others squash it.

RABBITS ARE OVERRUNNING YOUR HOUSE

Pet rabbits have come into the house. At first, you are entertained by their antics and feel affection for the fluffy little creatures. You then notice one doe has given birth to a litter of kittens; you enjoy the spectacle. But now there's a birth explosion—other doe rabbits have kittens as well. Instead of feeling indulgent, you get angry and start to pick up armfuls of rabbits to put them back outdoors where they live.

Action What are you doing in life that keeps doubling in number? Is spending money getting out of hand—are your debts, with increasing interest, mirroring those dozens of pet rabbits? If so, take this dream seriously. It started harmlessly enough and was even entertaining; then it got out of hand, escalating to the point of you being overwhelmed by the burden. Work on reining in your habit.

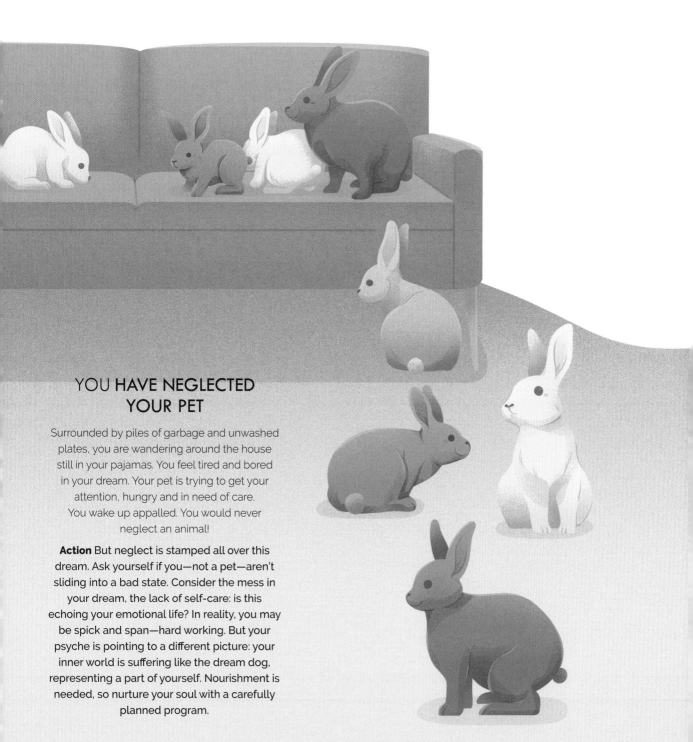

YOU HAVE NEGLECTED YOUR PET

Surrounded by piles of garbage and unwashed plates, you are wandering around the house still in your pajamas. You feel tired and bored in your dream. Your pet is trying to get your attention, hungry and in need of care. You wake up appalled. You would never neglect an animal!

Action But neglect is stamped all over this dream. Ask yourself if you—not a pet—aren't sliding into a bad state. Consider the mess in your dream, the lack of self-care: is this echoing your emotional life? In reality, you may be spick and span—hard working. But your psyche is pointing to a different picture: your inner world is suffering like the dream dog, representing a part of yourself. Nourishment is needed, so nurture your soul with a carefully planned program.

"

THE INTERPRETATION OF
DREAMS IS THE ROYAL
ROAD TO A KNOWLEDGE
OF THE UNCONSCIOUS.

"

SIGMUND FREUD
THE INTERPRETATION OF DREAMS

HORSES

Horses have been part of mankind's history. Beasts of burden, swift-footed travelers, agricultural workers—they have been essential companions throughout the centuries. Nowadays, they serve mostly for riding, their noble contribution to society outdated by technology, though horses have a newly recognized value in equine therapy. When they appear in dreams, they are potent symbols.

HORSES CHANGING COLOR

You are amazed at the sight of horses that seem to have the ability to change color on a whim, like a chameleon. You are full of wonder about how they can do this yet feel vaguely uncomfortable about their unpredictability.

Action There seems to be a warning here. What's unpredictable in your life currently? The images in the dream should offer meaning. If you think someone or a situation is one thing, they or it might prove to be entirely different. Trust is the issue: be watchful rather than believing everything you see. Being taken for a ride is not what you want!

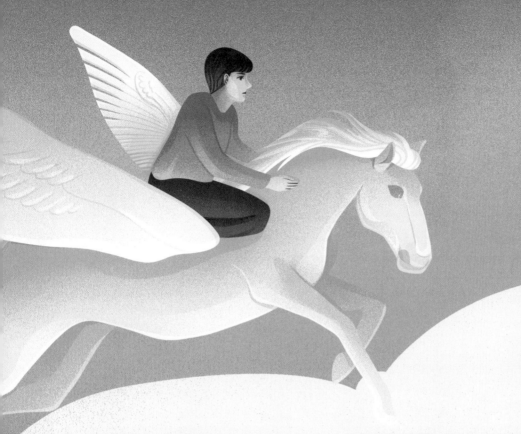

WINGING **THROUGH THE CLOUDS**

Riding bareback, you are on a magical horse flying through the clouds. It is beautiful up there in the sky, your mount dipping and diving in a glorious aerial ride. His feathered wings, like those of Pegasus, propel you both through the air. Joy fills you at the fun of the ride.

Action Take this dream as a spiritual message—a chance to glimpse a mystical world. Pegasus was made immortal for his loyalty and service; the god Zeus morphed him into a star. Consider yourself blessed to have ridden among the stars on this lovely horse. His message is one of encouragement for your down-to-earth efforts: he's acknowledging your daily struggle.

A **THRILLING HORSE RIDE**

You are mounted on a magnificent hunter horse, and you exult in the feeling of power under you. Your wonderful horse jumps effortlessly over gates and hedges. Your whole body tingles at the thrill of such power, and you are ecstatic about being carried away by the glory of this horse.

Action This is a sexual dream, primal in its energy and excitement. Are you the horse or the rider? Both can be true in the complexity of the dream world, but the dreamer is certainly lusting after a sexual encounter. Beware in real life, though, because making love with a partner may fall short of this. You could be accused of being too overbearing because you have abundant energy. Consider how best to channel it to enhance your love life.

WILD ANIMALS

They live in the jungle, on moors, in the savanna, and on the side of mountains. Untamed by humans, they roam as nature intended. In dreams, their killer instinct to survive appears symbolically to us from the depths of our inner world, where the socially unacceptable hides in the shadows.

ANGRY LIONS ROAR

Grazing animals raise their heads in alarm. You see a lion descending from his shady branch on a tree to investigate an intruder. A young male lion is about to invade the pride's space—a terrible fight ensues. You wake, still hearing their roars, and feel surprisingly angry yourself.

Action Dream the dream on: What happens next? Which wild animal survives—the old dominant lion or the hopeful young intruder? With which lion do you identify with and feel sympathy for? Consider that the lion is an instinctual part of yourself. Reflect on that anger and see how it mirrors episodes in your life where you may have wished to roar but instead kept quiet. Now face future challenges with a lion's courage.

WILD ANIMALS IN THE YARD

You are in an unknown house and notice through big windows that there are several pet animals in the yard. You go out to be friendly—and suddenly see these are no tame pets, but wild animals. Terrified, you flee back to the safety of the house, thankful to have realized this before anything worse happened.

Action Are you sometimes too trusting with people, offering yourself before you really get to know them? With the best of intentions, you go forward to be friendly, only to be disappointed later. Your psyche has illustrated your behavior pattern. Train yourself to size up more closely at first and identify potential danger before it could harm you.

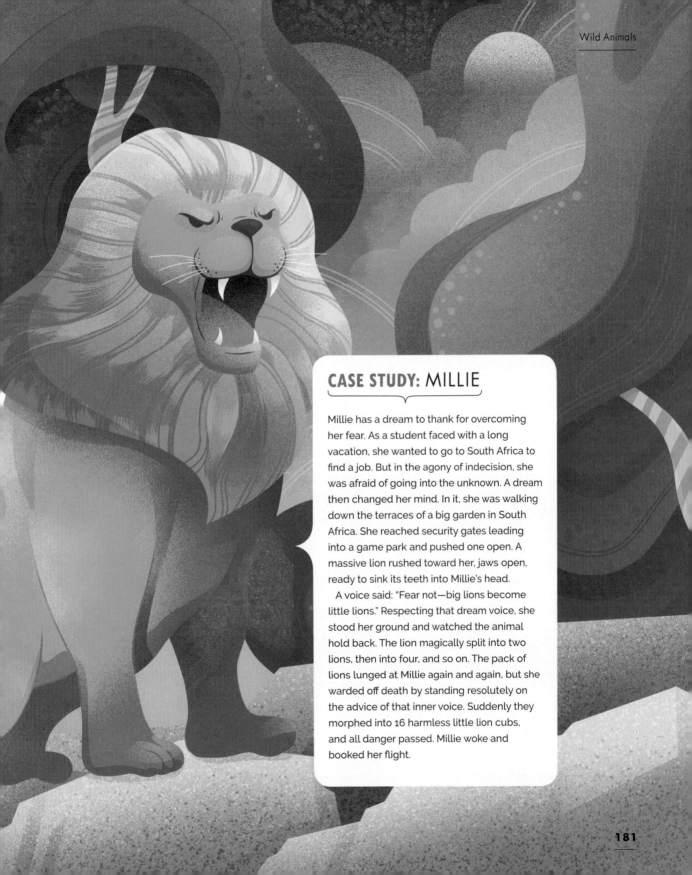

CASE STUDY: MILLIE

Millie has a dream to thank for overcoming her fear. As a student faced with a long vacation, she wanted to go to South Africa to find a job. But in the agony of indecision, she was afraid of going into the unknown. A dream then changed her mind. In it, she was walking down the terraces of a big garden in South Africa. She reached security gates leading into a game park and pushed one open. A massive lion rushed toward her, jaws open, ready to sink its teeth into Millie's head.

A voice said: "Fear not—big lions become little lions." Respecting that dream voice, she stood her ground and watched the animal hold back. The lion magically split into two lions, then into four, and so on. The pack of lions lunged at Millie again and again, but she warded off death by standing resolutely on the advice of that inner voice. Suddenly they morphed into 16 harmless little lion cubs, and all danger passed. Millie woke and booked her flight.

REPTILES

Reptiles, whether venomous or harmless, seldom rank as cuddly pets. They appear in our dreams as ancient messengers. Consider the snake's biblical role and its presence on the Rod of Asclepius, a symbol of medicine and healing. Reptiles can kill—or cure.

AN ALLIGATOR IN THE ROAD

You are walking down a lonely road, happy to be in the fresh air. You hear a rustle in the nearby bushes, imagining it to be a bird looking for worms. The rustling turns into a loud noise—horrifyingly, an alligator has jumped out and stares at you. It's clearly out of its comfort zone. You feel sorry for it.

Action Does this dream mirror your own emotions? Are you perhaps feeling inappropriately confined in a situation not conducive to a more natural existence? If it's not possible to make changes immediately, use this vivid dream to help you wait for and identify the right time to make your move.

A FORK-TONGUED MENACE

A giant monitor lizard is crashing his way along a path. His long, forked tongue is flickering menacingly as you watch him smell and locate his small prey. You are relieved to be off his path, so it's unlikely there will be a confrontation with the beast. But there's something uncomfortable about observing this big lizard.

Action The phrase "speaks with forked tongue" carries the implication of hypocrisy or deception. Are you are guilty of occasionally saying one thing but meaning another—if only to avoid hurting feelings? This sometimes seems justifiable, but it's not authentic. Consider the wisdom of gently speaking the truth, then there's no hidden agenda.

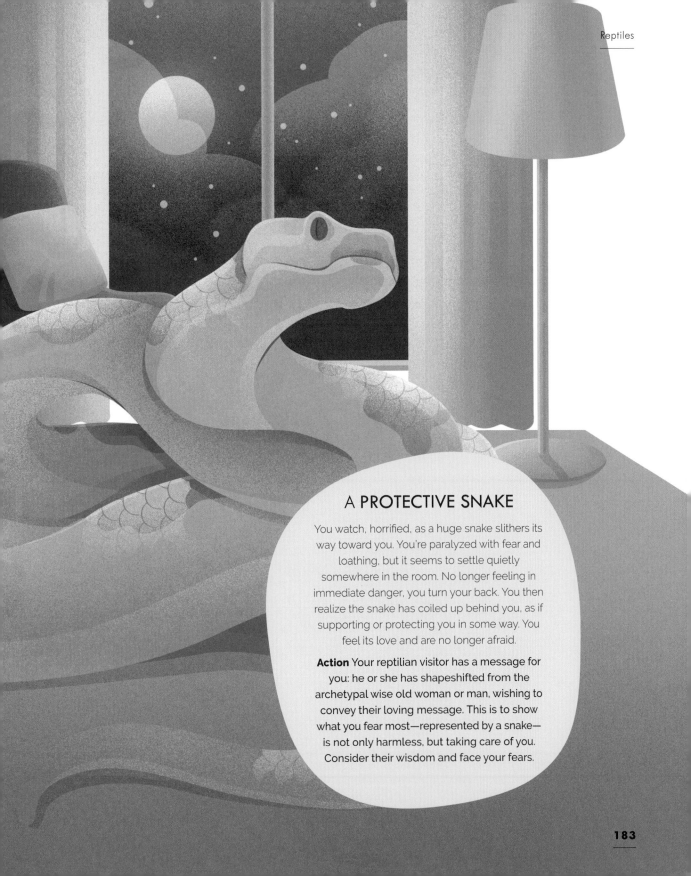

A PROTECTIVE SNAKE

You watch, horrified, as a huge snake slithers its way toward you. You're paralyzed with fear and loathing, but it seems to settle quietly somewhere in the room. No longer feeling in immediate danger, you turn your back. You then realize the snake has coiled up behind you, as if supporting or protecting you in some way. You feel its love and are no longer afraid.

Action Your reptilian visitor has a message for you: he or she has shapeshifted from the archetypal wise old woman or man, wishing to convey their loving message. This is to show what you fear most—represented by a snake— is not only harmless, but taking care of you. Consider their wisdom and face your fears.

183

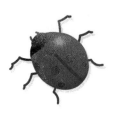

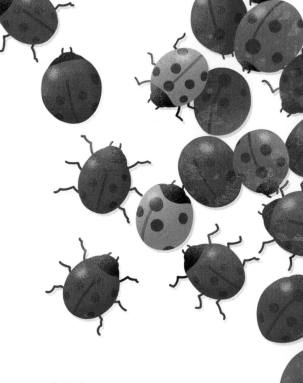

INSECTS

Insects are small animals, so it's surprising how much they are feared as creepy crawlies. They crop up in our dreams as species of all shapes and sizes yet, however harmless, they seem to remind us at a primal level of danger. Bites, stings, and invasion seem part of that ancient dread.

YOU WATCH A SPIDER POUNCE

In your dream, a giant spider comes out of its hiding place to investigate the silk web woven to trap its victim—and then waits in the shadows. It's a terrifying prospect, and you shudder to imagine the scene as its prey steps innocently into the silky trap. You then watch it played out: the spider pounces, pulling its prey down into its shadowy, dark hole.

Action Your psyche has used this unpleasant picture to help you begin to face either what has already happened to you in a real-life encounter or what you fear. Stalkers behave like the spider, as do sex offenders weaving silky, careful plans to get their wishes met. Don't be frightened by this dream; be grateful for it. Talk to a trusted friend or therapist.

YOU ARE BITTEN BY A TICK

Your dream takes you on a pleasant walk among tall grasses. The appearance later of a small tick on your thigh seems insignificant. Yet, as you watch, the tick grows larger and larger until it is full of your blood—so full, it balloons to the size of a basketball. It revolts you and yet you can't dislodge it. Somehow this reminds you of a recent emotion you've been experiencing.

Action Is there a psychological vampire draining you out there? Many people unwittingly steal your psychic energy, leaving you exhausted; others thrive unhealthily on taking from you. Realize the tick's bite is a metaphor for what's happening to you socially. Be more alert to the dangers: it's not a physical health hazard, but a mental or spiritual one. Choose your company carefully.

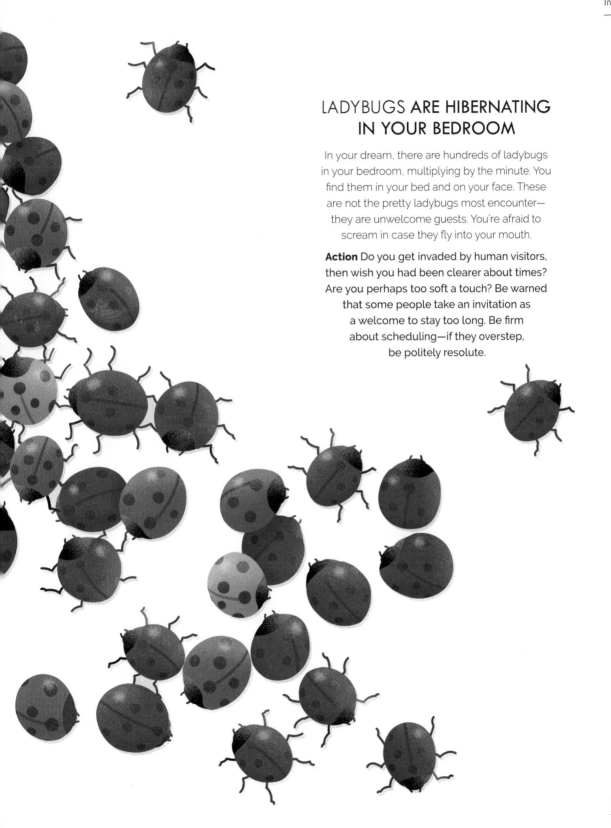

LADYBUGS ARE HIBERNATING IN YOUR BEDROOM

In your dream, there are hundreds of ladybugs in your bedroom, multiplying by the minute. You find them in your bed and on your face. These are not the pretty ladybugs most encounter—they are unwelcome guests. You're afraid to scream in case they fly into your mouth.

Action Do you get invaded by human visitors, then wish you had been clearer about times? Are you perhaps too soft a touch? Be warned that some people take an invitation as a welcome to stay too long. Be firm about scheduling—if they overstep, be politely resolute.

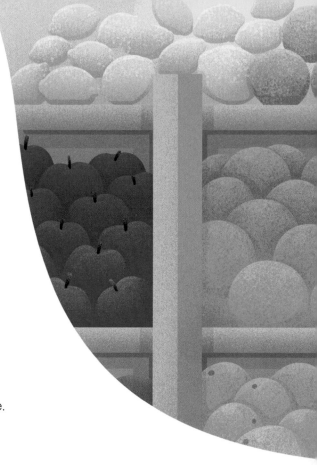

MAGGOTS IN FRUIT

Appearances can be deceiving in all manner of different guises, from succulent fruit to charming strangers. Whenever there's a possible hidden aspect to a seemingly good exterior, we need to be on red alert, if possible. Our dreams help by showing the reality of what is covert.

A STRANGER'S GIFT

A charming stranger is showing you a good deal of attention in the dream. They offer you ripe fruit as a gift, and you enjoy being the focus of their interest. You bite into the fruit and see a maggot inside. This unexpected shock corresponds now with the way the stranger seems to expect you to do something inappropriate. You feel wary.

Action You are right to be on guard. Remember, he or she could be you—or a part of you. What is it that you're hiding from yourself (and others) that you keep as well hidden as that maggot in the fruit? You may be failing to acknowledge the darker side of one of your subpersonalities. Being generous with gifts to win friendship, or whatever, has worked so far, but it's inauthentic. Your psyche is showing that it's time to work on owning that unacceptable part.

LATE SUMMER SCAVENGING

You and some friends are in an orchard in late summer. You're having so much fun in the dream finding fruit still on the trees—it doesn't feel like stealing, more like scavenging. Laughing, you all gather your little pile of fruit, knowing some will have maggots in them because it's end of season, but nobody cares.

Action This is a whimsical dream where you recaptured the fun of childhood and relished the joy of eating forbidden fruits—literally. Maggots, fungus, and bruised flesh are all part of the escapade: you eat or throw it away later. Is your psyche suggesting that you're being too responsible? That late season backdrop is a clue here. Being an adult holds so many "musts," perhaps you need to throw caution to the wind sometimes.

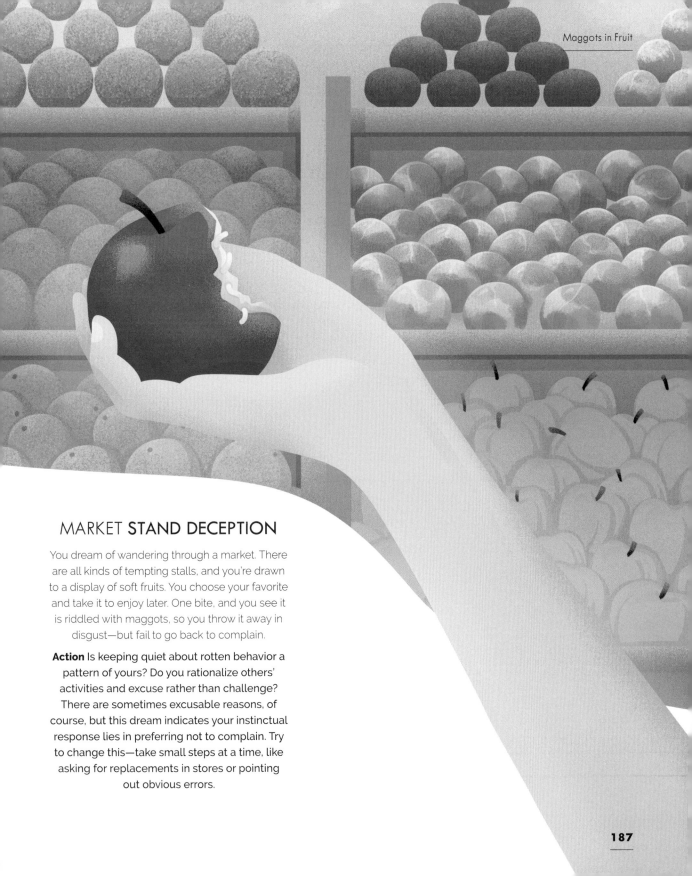

MARKET **STAND DECEPTION**

You dream of wandering through a market. There are all kinds of tempting stalls, and you're drawn to a display of soft fruits. You choose your favorite and take it to enjoy later. One bite, and you see it is riddled with maggots, so you throw it away in disgust—but fail to go back to complain.

Action Is keeping quiet about rotten behavior a pattern of yours? Do you rationalize others' activities and excuse rather than challenge? There are sometimes excusable reasons, of course, but this dream indicates your instinctual response lies in preferring not to complain. Try to change this—take small steps at a time, like asking for replacements in stores or pointing out obvious errors.

187

" DREAMS ARE TODAY'S ANSWERS TO TOMORROW'S QUESTIONS. "

EDGAR CAYCE

TREE FLOURISHING

The image of a beautiful canopy of leaves growing from a firm tree trunk and abundant branches easily summons memories of long summer days, the countryside, and happy times. Though dreaming of a tree in full leaf appears only positive, keep in mind that there may be other aspects in the scene pointing perhaps to more complex issues.

YOU ARE NOSTALGIC FOR TIMES PAST

The tree stands on its own, its splendor unappreciated because of its isolation. Nobody is around, and you feel wistful about its solitary state, You revisit your memories to gain comfort from better times in your life.

Action Accept those times are gone—let the nostalgia go while reminding yourself how rich those days were. As you, the dreamer, are the tree, acknowledge how it is flourishing despite the isolation. Seek new friends and create new memories.

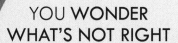

YOU WONDER WHAT'S NOT RIGHT

The landscape is bleak and makes you feel uneasy. You fear that the tree you see before you is planted in the wrong kind of soil—probably poor-quality earth. The tree has done its best to flourish against the odds, but it desperately needs nutrients and water.

Action As you are the tree here, consider how to start giving yourself more nourishment. You may have wasted time in a relationship or work situation, being drained and getting nothing back. Drastic change may not be necessary, but finding a means of replenishing your vital energies is.

YOU REJOICE TO SEE YOUR TREE FLOURISH

Your dream is full of good feeling. You are in a sunny place, warm with a sense of well-being. Your year may have held a difficult winter emotionally, but note that an abundant tree—particularly if it bears fruit—tells you the difficulties are either past or soon will be.

Action Congratulate yourself on having grown through whatever pain you endured. A fruitful tree—nature at her best—pinpoints healthy inner and outer world development.

YOU GRIEVE OVER A TREE'S LOSS

A branch has been sawn off a flourishing tree, and you are sad to see the imbalance. The dream shows sap oozing out of the wound—it's not yet healed over.

Action Is this mirroring something that happened to you, such as a loss or severance? Accept your emotional wound: tell yourself time and readjustment to the situation will eventually achieve release from the grief, whatever its cause.

UPROOTED TREE

There's something potentially sad about the image of an uprooted tree—it has become ungrounded, pulled from its safe home in the earth. However, in the dream world, there are other meanings to consider. Perhaps their appearance in your dream might suggest uprooting to a new home, career, or lifestyle.

MAKING ROOM FOR DEVELOPMENT

A large tree is about to be pulled down—arborists arrive, their noisy saws cutting through the top branches until the trunk is ready to be uprooted. Unmoved, you then feel surprisingly pleased as this majestic tree's roots and stump are finally pulled from the soil.

Action In the real world, people remove trees to make room for new development, or because they cast too much shadow. Is that what's happening in your inner life? Are you getting rid of emotional obstacles? If so, greet the changes—your feelings about the uprooted tree's disappearance suggest a positive outcome with no unpleasant surprises.

WINDS BLOW DOWN COUNTLESS TREES

You dream of a powerful wind uprooting trees and decimating woodland. There is nothing you can do but watch Mother Nature's fury destroy all that beauty. You imagine how birds and wildlife will have lost their habitat, and you're full of grief about such devastation.

Action Has a job loss, proposed change of location, or leaving familiar territory prompted this dream? A powerful wind would suggest events over which you have no control; there seems to be no opportunity available to fight off the impending change. You must go along with the new order.

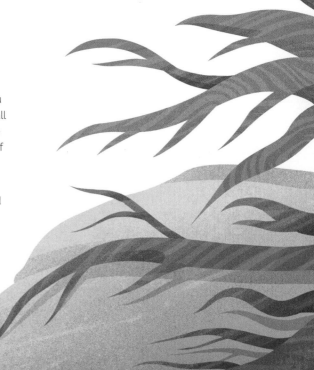

REARRANGING **THE LAYOUT**

You dream of watching someone digging up your favorite ornamental tree. At first, you're irritated at them for taking matters into their own hands. How dare they! You then realize how much better the uprooted tree will one day look, transplanted elsewhere in the park or yard and creating more visual balance.

Action Don't be afraid to initiate transitions instead of letting others do so. The dream tree could be a metaphor for yourself: passively submitting to others' plans. If it literally means transporting a favorite tree or bush to a new place, consider how good it will look after you've chosen exactly where you can transplant it. The same goes for your life. The key here is to do what you want (if possible), not watch others always make their choices.

CASE STUDY: KIERAN

Kieran had led a repressed life, living with a woman with poor self-esteem who needed to be the special one in the partnership. Their implicit collusive deal lasted for years, until he left her. He found a new job in landscape gardening—and Ella.

Ella was not into collusion, wanting an authentic man responsible for his own emotional development. Every time he fell back into the habitual self-effacing, she showed her angry frustration. Over time, Kieran began to understand why she was distressed at this suppression of his own needs. He learned to stand up for himself and to enjoy praise sincerely offered.

One night, a vivid dream confirmed how his psychological life was in the process of changing. He was pushing a wheelbarrow along a new road. The wheelbarrow was filled with rich soil into which an uprooted tree had been placed, ready for planting. He understood that he was that tree—ready now to flourish and grow in very different soil from the bleak territory he had once thought acceptable.

ROTTING FRUIT

It's a sad day when what was once new and wholesome gets left unwanted and slowly rots. This applies not only to fruit: anything grown from seed that goes unappreciated and ignored is being denied its destiny. Dreams can tell us more.

PILES OF UNWANTED FRUITS

There are heaps of apples and pears left to rot. You find the sight distressing, thinking of the people who might have welcomed these unwanted goods before they were inedible. Someone then appears in the dream and shovels piles of the fruit into a container: so they do want it! You realize that rotting fruit has a purpose—perhaps to add to a compost heap or to feed birds in winter.

Action Never assume! Your dream is showing you that first impressions are not necessarily the right ones. That pile of unwanted fruit had a planned future, but not as you imagined it. Can you link this observation to events in your life? If assuming first and being surprised later is a pattern of yours, correct this instinctive habit. It keeps you from seeing the bigger picture.

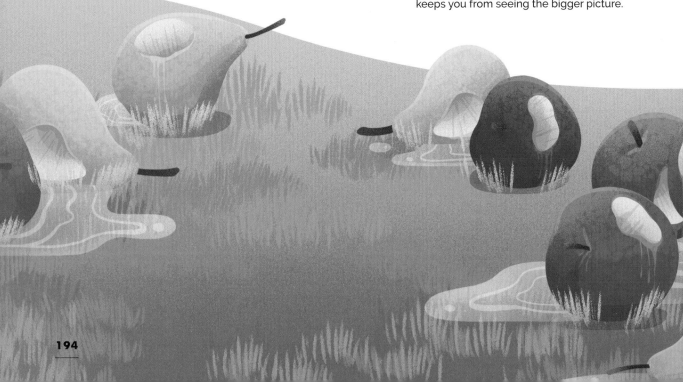

PAST **THEIR SELL-BY DATE**

You dream of a group of beautiful women visiting a market. One pauses by a fruit stand. Suddenly, she calls to her companions that the fruit here is overripe, well past its sell-by date. She's warning them against buying what she insists is rotting produce, despite the stand worker's angry denial. You notice she looks upset and worried rather than displeased. You feel sorry for her, realizing the fruit is not the real reason for her distress.

Action Can you identify with this woman? Do you fear that you're reaching your sell-by date in looks? Take a hint from the feelings in your dream. You were sad to witness her emotional response to the fruit she called rotten—she was transferring her feelings about herself onto the freshly picked market produce. Your psyche is showing you that people get frightened about not looking good enough. Accept it's what you are that counts.

AN **ANGRY MOB THROWS ROTTEN FRUIT**

Men and women hold protest signs, and you edge forward to see what's going on. It looks like a political meeting: key people arrive to take up their places. Someone then throws rotten tomatoes at several of them. Those at whom the rotten fruits are hurled are surprisingly unruffled. You feel sorry for their plight yet somehow know they feel the aggressive act was justified.

Action If you are currently angry about recent unfair behavior, consider what this dream is underlining: you want to show your disgust in a disgusting manner. But the victims take their punishment without reacting furiously. Try confronting whoever treated you unfairly, but use calm words only—and wait to see if the dream message isn't played out in their response, your anger and their guilt respectively resolved.

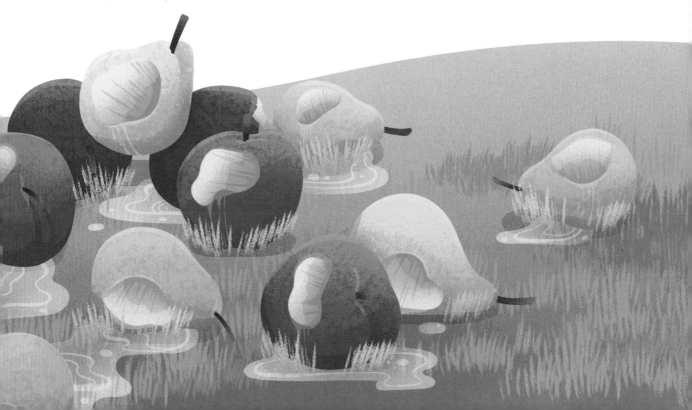

VOLCANO ERUPTING

A volcano's deep-down pool of molten rock is usually dormant. But when it erupts, the fallout is violent and potentially dangerous. There's a parallel here with angry people's behavior: tempers erupt fiercely and can be just as unpredictable. Dreams can often help warn of their arrival.

YOU ARE ESCAPING THE LAVA

You hear a rumbling sound, then screams of terrified people as a volcano erupts. In the dream, you run with all the others to try to escape the red-hot lava flow. Instinctively, you go in the opposite direction the lava takes, sensing you're on the right path. It seems to lead to safer ground.

Action Is an eruption about to happen in your life? If you have to make a decision about a major life change, keep in mind how that is going to affect others as they struggle with the difficult fallout. You need to prepare those around you and warn them to keep their distance as you deal with your personal red-hot challenge.

A **VOLCANO HAS KILLED PEOPLE**

You dream of walking through the streets in a community below a volcano, where the bodies of countless people are strewn everywhere. It's as if they died in seconds while they were going about their daily business. You then realize their deaths were caused by the volcano's poisonous gases. The scene is eerie and very troubling.

Action Are you afraid of sudden calamity happening to you and your family? Some trigger (tales of Vesuvius?) created this dream, but its message could have come from any source. The need here is to accept that tragedy happens. But there is no more reason for it to happen to you and yours than to anyone—it's important to take a view that life is to be enjoyed now, come what may.

VOLCANIC **DISRUPTION**

Your bags are packed, tickets and passport safely in hand for the flight to your vacation. Suddenly you hear news of a volcanic eruption that somehow stops you from flying to your destination. You are devastated. How could so unexpected an event put an end to your longed-for break? You angrily feel like something should be done about these natural disasters: politicians or clever scientists should be able to control them.

Action Not only is this unreasonable, it's impossible: nature rules. Are you feeling angry with people closer to home, resentful that actions haven't been taken to make your life easier? Think about taking some power yourself, not leaving it to others to improve a situation.

DROWNING

Water is found all over the earth. It visually manifests in beautiful rivers, oceans, streams, lakes, and solid ice. It keeps us alive—and yet it can be the cause of our death should we either have too much or too little of it. Small wonder dreams show us water in all its power.

DROWNING IN DESPAIR

Against a backdrop rather like a watery grave, there's no actual storyline to this dream. Its impact comes with a depressive quality lurking in the depths—you're somehow all alone underwater. There's a sense of nearly drowning in it, yet in the dream you know this is not the end.

Action Depression presents in all shades of gray, and the dream shows simply how you see yourself today. If that view goes on too long, contact your doctor to discuss if medication is the best way forward. If your state of mind would seem better addressed by therapy or counseling, make an appointment to get started.

NEWBORN ANIMALS ARE DROWNED

Someone has told you some newborn animals are going to be drowned. You're assured it's the kindest way to get rid of them because nobody will want to care for them. You are sad at the thought and want to save those little creatures, defenseless as they are.

Action These helpless newborn animals are metaphors for some part of you that feels unwanted. A subpersonality identifies with them being powerless to resist their fate, as your dreaming self believes them to be. Notice you don't actually see them being drowned—you only gather that this is planned. So address your phobia that you're not wanted: you need to check out what the situation is in reality. Try some straight talk—ask your employer, partner, or friend how they feel about your relationship. If for any reason their answer implies it's time to move on, be thankful your dream nudged you to dispel the impasse.

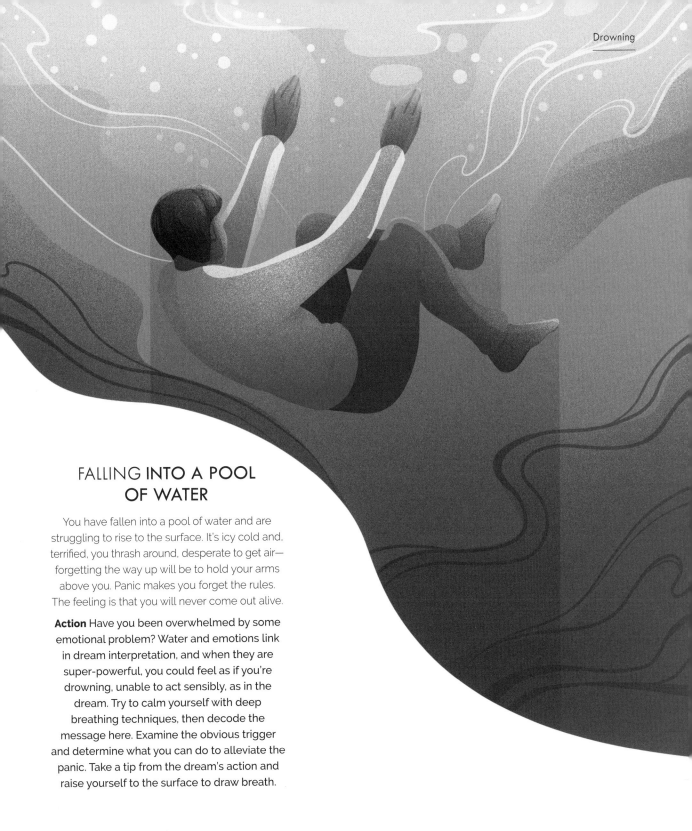

FALLING INTO A POOL OF WATER

You have fallen into a pool of water and are struggling to rise to the surface. It's icy cold and, terrified, you thrash around, desperate to get air—forgetting the way up will be to hold your arms above you. Panic makes you forget the rules. The feeling is that you will never come out alive.

Action Have you been overwhelmed by some emotional problem? Water and emotions link in dream interpretation, and when they are super-powerful, you could feel as if you're drowning, unable to act sensibly, as in the dream. Try to calm yourself with deep breathing techniques, then decode the message here. Examine the obvious trigger and determine what you can do to alleviate the panic. Take a tip from the dream's action and raise yourself to the surface to draw breath.

SWIMMING IN THE OCEAN

There's something seductive about sinking into a warm ocean—it's like a continuation of the safe confines of the womb, or luxuriating in the pleasure of a hot bath. But the ocean has even greater charm, perhaps because of its vastness; there's more freedom to move. It's a familiar setting for dreams.

SWIMMING **NAKED**

You dream of stripping off your clothes and running to the water's edge. Another person has had the same thought, and together you meet and swim in a gloriously warm ocean. Skin-to-skin contact follows, though there is nothing sexual about it—just two people rejoicing in the freedom of this wonderful day. You feel entirely comfortable; it's like being with an old and loved friend.

Action This is about reconnecting with a loved one. Here, the second bather is your *animus* or your *anima* (depending on your own gender)—the other half that makes you whole. Water represents our emotional life, so this is a positive dream in a beautiful, warm setting. You have reunited with the missing part of yourself!

A **SENSUAL FROLIC**

It's a warm, sultry night, and in the dream you're floating on your back in the ocean looking up at the stars. Friends are splashing around nearby, not looking up at the stars—they are having too much fun to notice them. While the scene is perfect, something is lacking for you to feel happy. Someone then swims up to you, and you make sensual love in the warm ocean. Now you lack for nothing.

Action A wishful scenario that's healthy and right: you seem to have been feeling outside the mainstream of activity in your life (note looking upward rather than toward your friends), and the isolation has its pathos. Think of planning a vacation if you can—somewhere to enjoy the warm ocean—and the rest will take care of itself. If that's not possible, turn toward your friends anyway and somehow make yourself slightly less of an outsider.

CHILDREN **SWIMMING**

Children are paddling in the shallow waters, and you notice one or two venturing too far out for safety. The warmth of the seawater keeps them happily immersed for hours—but as an onlooker, you begin to worry about them. Somehow there are fewer children than you first noticed. Where have they gone? Are they in danger? Have they drowned? You panic and wake up tense with fear.

Action Do you tend to feel overly concerned for others, when they should be looking after their own responsibilities? That increasing worry in the dream suggests you need to check your anxieties about general issues in your own life; you've projected those anxieties onto unknown children. Identify yourself as one of them—a young part of you that always felt helpless to stop bad things from happening.

A SUBMERGED VESSEL

Whatever lies underwater carries the hidden allure of the unknown: that which is beneath the waves has mystery because it's unseen. In Jungian terms, when we contemplate what is below the surface, we address the unconscious. Our dreaming self thrives on the symbolism.

SHIPWRECK IN A FAKE OCEAN

You watch in horror as a boat flounders and sinks, slowly disappearing beneath the water like it would in a wartime disaster movie. You realize this is a movie, all pretense, and nobody is in danger. Your dream then shows other similar scenes with fake high drama, with stuntmen performing the dangerous parts. Waking, you reflect on the cleverness of illusion.

Action Is there a parallel running in your life where apparent disaster is only a facade? Your unconscious is offering a warning: learn to investigate what's "under the water," and don't risk being fooled by appearances.

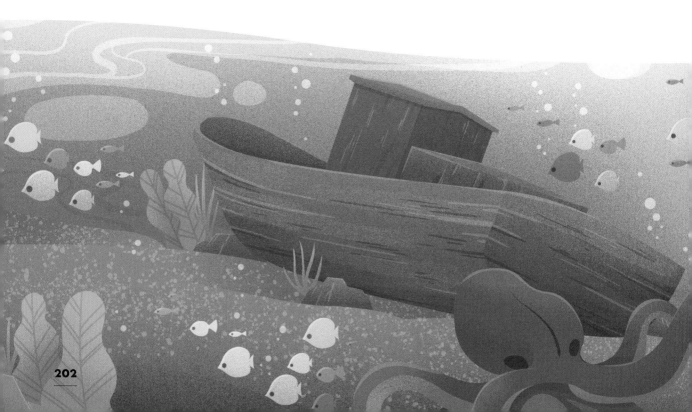

A MYSTERIOUS VESSEL

Someone has indicated a vessel has been thrown into the water, but it's lost. They are concerned about it—is it valuable?—and you desperately want to find it. You dive down into the dark water to try to retrieve whatever it is and, more importantly, what it might contain. The water is dark and threatening, but you glimpse something.

Action Your psyche is hinting at the need for self-exploration, perhaps by going into therapy. Diving down into the unconscious is part of the work: the need is to find the metaphorical vessel submerged in your inner world that holds the answers to much of your unhappiness. Reflect first on what it might contain—submerged painful memories?—then consider finding the right therapist.

SUBMERGED TOY BOATS

Tide pools on a familiar beach recall childhood vacations, with all the stuff like buckets and spades. You then see, submerged in the bottom of one pool, replica toys of real boats you once sailed in. You pull one out of its hideaway, feeling emotional.

Action What particular memories do these toys hold for you? Is there an anniversary or event in your life currently resonating with this dream? Identify them and see if they relate with this activity, or the emotional content about the anniversary. Useful insight could come from contemplating the authentic feelings associated with the dream toys.

CASE STUDY: DYLAN

Dylan had been a timid schoolboy and left school without qualifications to drift into a boring job. His innate intelligence had gone unnoticed until one day he found himself talking at the bus stop with a retired professor.

Their conversation excited Dylan and led him to search out books on the subject they had discussed. Next time he met the professor, their meeting resulted in him being encouraged to study part time at the local college. His whole outlook changed as, steered by his concerned new friend, he went on to take tests and find a fulfilling job.

One night, he dreamed of watching a huge Viking longboat being hauled up out of the water. He knew the boat was a metaphor for himself: sunk without a trace for so long but now brought to the surface. There was an old man with a beard standing by in the dream—his senex, or wise man—and he knew he had the professor (as a living wise man) to thank for nudging him toward reaching his apt potential.

TSUNAMIS AND FLOODS

A tsunami can carry a crucial message in dreams, symbolically showing the scale of emotional turbulence experienced by the dreamer. We know seismic ocean waves are a source of great danger, terrifying in their force and unpredictability. Day-to-day crises can seem in our sleep just like the hugeness of those giant waves.

LEARNING TO FACE THE WAVES

You see a tsunami coming toward you in the dream and hold tightly to a strong support. The wave gets closer and closer—you grip firmly and duck your head down to take the crashing water. It hurtles over you and moves on. You're safe.

Action Despite day-to-day turbulence—water being linked to emotions—you show resilience in this dream. Meditating on the reason you feel a "tsunami" is out to get you would be a good plan. Has life knocked you around too much? Have you felt near drowning emotionally? Recall your inner strength. The dream tells you clearly about survival—trust it.

FLOODWATERS
SURROUND YOU

Floodwater surrounds where you live. The dream shows you no obvious route to dry land, and you fear being helpless to move, cut off from other people. As the water seeps into the ground floor, you decide to climb the stairs or somehow get on to the roof. From there, you see rescue activity going on and realize it's only a matter of patiently waiting your turn.

Action The flood is a metaphor for you feeling powerless to move. Without the necessary equipment—resources, money, time—you are being shown that waiting patiently is your only option. Floodwater always subsides, so take it to mean that what surrounds you now—emotional stress, overwork, family worries—will seep away.

A TSUNAMI DESTROYS

You dream of a devastating tsunami destroying everything in its path once the wave hits land. There is a scene of complete destruction, nothing left on which to build a new life.

Action Is this reflecting your own thoughts about emotional life destroying you now? If you feel there's nothing left on which to build a new life, see the positive message implicit here. You must move on, consider change, and build a different environment for yourself. If the equivalent of a tsunami had not struck you, think of how fixed you might have remained. Your dream is urging you to leave the untenable.

"

EVERYONE CAN DERIVE
IMMEASURABLE BENEFITS
FROM LOOKING INTO
THE WORLD OF HIS OWN
SYMBOLOGY.

"

KEVIN J. TODESCHI
DREAM IMAGES AND SYMBOLS

GLOSSARY

These are some of the common terms used in psychotherapy relating to dream interpretation that have been used in this book.

ANIMA/ANIMUS

The *anima* and *animus* represent the unconscious sides to a man or woman, respectively: the *animus* is the unconscious masculine side of a woman and the *anima* the feminine side of a man. When a person has achieved a union of those two sides within their inner world, they reach a balanced state.

ARCHETYPE

The heroes and gods of the Greek pantheon gave Carl Jung the idea for his theory of archetypes—models of people, personalities, and ways of behaving that resonate with what we hear about the mythical characters from that ancient world. When present-day people behave with certain clearly defined characteristics—for example, the hero who rushes to rescue those in distress—they are playing out a primordial, universal role, or an inborn tendency cultivated in his or her upbringing to get them through life as easily as possible. There are many archetypes, but to mention a few here, we have the Trickster, the Warrior, the Mother, the Thief, the Fool, the Magician, and the Prostitute (not to be confused with sex workers; it's more about the qualities of discounting one's personal value, such as people "prostituting" their art by performing lesser functions).

CONSCIOUSNESS

In lay terms, consciousness means that the waking self is aware of experiences constantly changing and shifting as it functions according to feelings, reactions, and social and parental conditioning. When hidden psychological material surfaces to the conscious mind—usually through the therapeutic process—that significance can and should be embraced and integrated into the person's conscious process, thus bringing the unknown into consciousness.

GRANDIOSITY

This describes a puffed-up sense of self—an unrealistic sense of superiority where a person believes themselves to be better than others. Grandiosity is seen clinically as part of a narcissistic personality disorder, where low self-esteem is central to that condition. Yet this unrealistic sense of self can apply to anyone where, for example, a dream reveals a hidden longing to be special, such as being friends with royalty or with celebrities. This does not necessarily indicate a disorder, more an unconscious need to be, or identify with being, important.

HUBRIS

This is an exaggerated self-confidence born of self-delusion—a belief that we have much to be proud about. It often manifests as arrogance. Our dreams sometimes help point this out; the challenge then is to heed the clues.

INDIVIDUATION

This is the path to the center, as Carl Jung describes the process, in which the individual becomes distinct—where we become an independent, separate entity. The balance between the unconscious and conscious mind has been achieved to become totally integrated as a person. When you have achieved individuation, you are no longer functioning from received ways of looking at life—learned from our parents or cultural environment—but from an authentic sense of self. At this point, it can be said that we have psychologically grown up.

INFLATION

Similar to hubris, this is a description in psychotherapeutic terms of being self-important. This is often compensating for feeling unimportant or inferior. Imagine pumping oneself up like a tire, or as a male bird does to look dominant. That comparative hugeness is imposing if we present ourselves to the world with this large (false) personality.

INNER WORLD

Having an inner and outer world is common to us all. The inner world is distinct from the outer, for it's within that psychological region we meet our emotional life, our spiritual selves, and—in a sense—where our psyche (or soul) presides. Our dreams will be created here, their presentation forged by the psyche that knows so much more than we do in the outer world, where the ego presides. The **OUTER WORLD** is the place of existence, where we make relationships, build a career, and take on responsibility. Meditation is said to help create balance between the two worlds.

METAPHOR

This is a figure of speech where a word—or action—refers to one thing (not literally applicable) by mentioning another. For example, a man might be described as being a pillar of the community. Obviously that can't be true, but it conveys a sense of that man's presence or uprightness in his community. Metaphors appear in dreams more often than not, perhaps because they so usefully sum up the psyche's meaning. As another example, a long object could be a penis (if we follow Sigmund Freud's thinking); a house signifies the dreamer, with its basement representing the unconscious, hidden aspects and the attic those issues that are related to the mind, the brain, or with spiritual matters. As we learn from the dream content, decoding this will depend on the setting, the felt sense, people, and the narrative.

PERSONA

Originally a persona was a mask used by actors: nowadays, the word describes the psychological mask many—if not most—people wear to hide their real selves. This is not a bad thing, nor is it duplicitous. It helps people feel more comfortable, just as cosmetics or a new suit can make the wearer feel more confident when they present themselves to the world. Used in psychological terms, persona means an aspect of character that is deliberately (or unintentionally) presented. For example, the comedian of the party can in reality be a very unhappy person.

PROJECTION

This applies to anyone who disowns some aspect of themselves they are probably uncomfortable with and project that quality onto another person. Dreams can sometimes illustrate this by showing the dreamer someone else's behavior as over-the-top outrageous, yet it resonates with how the dreamer secretly feels sometimes about themselves in real life. It's as if they are being nudged into a better understanding of what they do when awake. Many couples use projection without realizing it or the harm it causes. They hurl angry words at the other when their anger should have been expressed long ago, perhaps to a mother, father, teacher, or sibling. But children were taught not to, or punished if they showed their fury at the appropriate time, so the pent-up rage has been suppressed for years—and a partner gets the full brunt of it.

PSYCHE

The psyche is the totality of the human mind, conscious and unconscious. Carl Jung believed that the psyche works to regulate the system; we can see this happening through the psyche's presentation of helpful dreams to encourage internal balance. The psyche has also been described as the human soul, mind, or spirit.

SHADOW

Just as the name suggests, that which has not been illuminated is cast into the shadows. This applies to unfavorable, disliked aspects of ourselves (self-determined) that we keep well hidden for obvious reasons. The shadow is the unacknowledged aspect of the self deemed unacceptable or too frightening to bring out into the light. People's shadow side appears when events prompt unguarded

GLOSSARY CONTINUED

responses, such as irritation or violent reaction, before it can be reined in.

SUBPERSONALITY

A subpersonality is a split-off part of the inner world's main characters, usually regarded as unacceptable or embarrassing. Similar to the archetypes, we carry within us many subpersonalities—perhaps a judge, a joker, even a potential murderer—all locked away within that world for fear of them compromising difficult situations in life. People speak of being "taken over" by some part of themselves they didn't know existed: it does.

Through habit, we usually hide the unacceptable or unsocial subpersonalities, but one can pop out when least expected, maybe triggered by a current situation. It's best to try to identify them early, if possible, to recognize what might be happening when they emerge.

SYMBOLS

The dreaming self uses symbols to state the obvious: you see a bridge and it means crossing to the other side; a letter brings news; a policeman represents law and order; a wallet signifies money or your identity; or a train takes you from one place to another, implicating travel or a journey. An entire dream could be said to present itself in symbols.

FURTHER READING

Largely influenced by Carl Jung's approach, this book focuses on metaphors and symbols, the spiritual and archetypes. If you wish to continue your journey with dream interpretation, the following books make for interesting additional reading:

Why We Sleep Matthew Walker (Penguin Random House UK, 2018)

Focusing Eugene Gendlin (Rider, an imprint of Ebury Publishing, 2003)

Mindfulness Bhante Henepola Gunaratana (Wisdom Publications, 2002)

Why Can't I Meditate? Nigel Wellings (Penguin Random House, 2015)

Inner Work Robert A. Johnson (Harper Collins, 1989)

Dreams That Change Our Lives Robert J. Hoss and Robert P. Gongloff, Editors (Chiron Publications Asheville North Carolina, 2017)

The Essential Jung Selected writings introduced by Anthony Storr (Fontana Press, 1983)

Memories, Dreams, Reflections Carl Jung (Fontana Press, 1995)

The Biology of Belief Bruce Lipton (Hay House UK Ltd., 2015)

There is a River: The story of Edgar Cayce Thomas Sugrue (A .R. E. Press, Virginia Beach, 1997)

Dream Images and Symbols Kevin J. Todeschi (A .R. E. Press, Virginia Beach, 1995)

PSYCHOTHERAPY WEBSITES

American Counseling Association
counseling.org

The world's largest organization representing professional counselors of various practice types.

United States Association for Body Psychotherapy (USABP)
usabp.org

A professional organization supporting the practice of somatic/body psychotherapy that believes memory is held in the body and can be retrieved.

International Psychotherapy Institute
theipi.org

Provides psychotherapy certification training programs for mental health professionals.

American Psychological Association
apa.org

Includes information on what psychotherapy is, plus how to find a psychologist undergoing psychotherapy.

Very Well Mind
verywellmind.com

Search for "psychotherapy" on their website to learn more about your options for treatment.

The Society of Analytical Psychology
thesap.org.uk

A professional body for Jungian analysts and psychotherapists that offers psychotherapy and analysis.

SOURCES

Why Do We Dream?
Matthew Walker, *Why We Sleep,*
Penguin Random House UK, 2018

Ibid. Rapid Eye Movement (REM) and Non-Rapid Eye
Movement (NREM)

Michael J. Breus, "Why Do We Dream?" [web article],
February 2015 https://www.thesleepdoctor.com.
Psychology Today https:///www.psychologytoday.
com/gb sleep-newzzz/201502/why-do-we-dream

What is Healthy Sleep?
J. L. Kavanau, "Sleep, memory maintenance, and
mental disorders," *Journal of Neuropathy* and C*linical
Neurosciences.* 12 (2): 199-208

Michelle Carr, "What's Behind Your Recurring
Dreams" [web article], *Psychology Today*
https://www.psychologytoday.com/gb/blog/
dream-factory/201411/
whats-behind-your-recurring-dreams

Lee Ann Obringer, "*How Dreams Work"* [web article],
https://science.howstuffworks.com/life/
inside-the-mind/human-brain/dreams8.htm.
Retrieved July 26, 2018

National Sleep Foundation, https://sleepfoundation.
org/sleep-topics/what-circadian-rhythmn

Massachusetts Institute of Technology
Animals have complex dreams, MIT researcher proves.
Retrieved July 26, 2018

The Dream Pioneers
Sigmund Freud, *The Interpretation of Dreams,*
Macmillan, translated by A. A. Brill, 1913

Anthony Storr, *The Essential Jung* Selected Writings,
Fontana Press, 1998

Calvin S. Hall, *The Meaning of Dreams,*
Harper & Brothers, New York, 1953

Edgar Casey, Kevin J. Todeschi, *Dream Images and
Symbols*, Creative Breakthroughs Inc., 1995

Dream Interpretation Through the Ages
"Ancient Theories About Dreams" [web article],
uploaded by Carla Barbe http://www.academia.
edu/3100958

"Chinese Dream Interpretation" [web article],
http://dreaming.life/interpreting-dreams/
ancient-chinese-dream-interpretation.htm

"Ancient History Encyclopedia" [web article],
http://ancient.eu/Akhenaten

"Dreams and Visions of God" [web article],
http://www.wpcdurham.org/
joseph-dreams-and-visions-of-god/

"The Legend of Yorkshire's Famous Prophetess"
[web article], http://yorkshirepost.co.uk
http://en.wikipedia.org/wiki/Nostradamus

Precognitive Dreams
Freud Museum, "The Interpretation of Dreams" [web
article], 1899, https://freud.org.uk/learn/discover-
psychoanalysis/the-interpretation-of-dreams/

Carl Jung, *Memories, Dreams, Reflections,* Random
House Inc., 1961

"Remote Viewing" [web article],
https://en.wikipedia.org/wiki/RemoteViewing

"Prophetic Dreams" [web article], https://www.
dream-interpretation.org.uk/types-of-dreams/
prophetic-dreams-htm

Rebecca Turner, "World of Lucid Dreaming" [web
article], https://www.world-of-lucid-dreaming.
com/10-dreams-that-changed-the-course-of-
human-history.html

Lucid Dreaming
Lee Ann Obringer, [web article], https://science.
howstuffworks.com/life/inside/the mind/
human-brain/dreams8.htm

Stephen Laberge *Lucid Dreaming* (excerpt with
Jeffrey Mishlove)—*A Thinking Allowed*—[online video],

https://www.youtube.com/watch?v=IG-sDcQiqMI
August 28, 2010

Secondary sources
Stanley Krippner (Foreword), Robert J. Hoss, & Robert P. Gongloff, editors, *Dreams That Change Our Lives*, Chiron Publications, 2017

Eugene T. Gendlin, *Focusing*, Penguin Random House Group, 2003

Bhante Henepola Gunaratana, *Mindfulness In Plain English*, Wisdom Publications, Boston, 2002

Robert A. Johnson, *Inner Work*, HarperCollins Publishers, 1989

COUNSELING AND PSYCHOTHERAPY

Sometimes recurring dreams, nightmares, or even intriguingly similar storylines that keep cropping up could indicate that finding help beyond this book might be worth considering. Many people can feel confused, distressed, or just plain curious without realizing they are unconsciously struggling with unresolved issues. Talking to a professional therapist or counselor could prove useful in the search for more clarity.

What is the difference between therapy and counseling? In the broadest terms, counselors work with the material their clients bring in the here and now and usually work on a shorter time frame than their more extensively trained colleagues in psychotherapy. By definition, the latter suggests longer and deeper work in practice, as the therapist explores hidden areas of trauma (however slight, childhood disappointment can still leave scars), bringing to the surface repressed, hurt feelings about which the conscious mind is unaware.

It's been said that counselors address the conscious mind, while psychotherapists look to the unconscious mind for their answers. This is not to disparage the valuable work achieved in the briefer encounters—more to explain what to expect if you

decide to go ahead and explore your material with a trained psychotherapist.

However, when troubling or fascinating dreams seem to encourage more insight than this book can offer, it might be preferable to consult the specialists whose training will have included some understanding of the vast subject of the unconscious mind. National directories will provide names and qualifications you will need (see page 211 for details of professional bodies). Always inquire if dreams are of special interest to a prospective practitioner.

If signing up for sessions in talk therapy does not appeal, consider contacting an accredited organization. It's possible that someone local (for example, a Jungian Analyst) might themselves be interested in teaching dream interpretation. Find out if that person would be prepared to run workshops on the subject. Under experienced professional guidance, you would discover the group's input both fascinating and revealing. This could surely be the start of a psychological journey to treasure.

INDEX

ABOUT THE AUTHOR

Rosie March-Smith, UKCP, BCPC, and Member Emeritus of the UK Association of Humanistic Psychology Practitioners, has been a psychotherapist for nearly 30 years. She began her working life as a newspaper journalist and ultimately became a freelance international feature writer. A tutor in Creative Writing at Denman College, Oxon, England, and other UK colleges of Further Education, she also taught prisoners in Reading Gaol, where the playwright Oscar Wilde was once imprisoned.

An increasing interest in the psychology (and hidden distress) lying behind her students' written work spurred her to train as a psychotherapist. For over a decade, she ran residential holistic living workshops in tandem with creative writing from her home in Somerset, England, where she still lives.

Rosie was a co-founder of The Dorset Association of Counselling and Psychotherapy, which offers speakers, workshops, and support to professional therapists from all over the West Country.

She is also the author of two Open University Press publications—*Counselling Skills for Complementary Therapists* and *Relationship Therapy* (McGraw-Hill Education).

ACKNOWLEDGMENTS

Author's acknowledgments
The author would like to thank colleagues Jo Lacy Smith, Julia Penrose, Molly Sobey, Flora Myer, Frances Hatch, Thekla Hickman, Sam Carr, and Derek Smith for their invaluable help in research and providing enthusiastic support. Jungian Analyst Matthew Harwood inspired a particular interest in dream work over the years with his study group: heartfelt gratitude for his time, interest, and intuitive insights.

Thanks are also due to James March-Smith and Mathew March-Smith for their unfailing response to correct computer queries as and when they cropped up on the author's unpredictable machine. Pong Cheese must be thanked for helpful information on the effect of cheese on dreams, good or bad, according to the nutritional value of the variety.

Many of the case studies were offered by clients past and present, all of whom gladly gave their permission for inclusion in this book; thanks are most certainly due to them.

Finally, the publisher's editor Emma Hill made the entire project not only smooth but greatly enjoyable—the author offers the warmest of thanks for her patience and gentle encouragement throughout.

Publisher's acknowledgments
DK would like to thank Matthew Bowes for his work on the early structuring of this book, John Friend for proofreading, and Marie Lorimer for the index.